Nature
the only
Healer

ACHARYA S. SWAMINATHAN

wisdom
tree

© S. Swaminathan, 2005

First published 2005
Reprinted 2006, March 2007, March 2009

ISBN 81-8328-009-9

Published by
Wisdom Tree
4779/23 Ansari Road
Darya Ganj, New Delhi-110002
Ph.: 23247966/67/68

Published by Shobit Arya for Wisdom Tree; *copy edited by* Manju Gupta; *designed by* Kamal
P. Jammual; *typeset at* Marks & Strokes, New Delhi –110002 and *printed at* Print Perfect, New
Delhi -110064

Dedicated to
Acharya Lakshmana Sarma

Contents

Preface

Back in the 19th century, Reverend Father Sebestian Kneipp had stated that all disease is but tissue uncleanliness.

How to restore the tissue cleanliness within and how to live in tune with the laws of personal hygiene leading to a radical cure of even the so-called incurable diseases are vital topics to be known to every person in the world. It is this that forms the core of this treatise, which is equally important for the healthy too who, by treading the path set herein, can prevent the onset of diseases like high or low blood pressure, diabetes, hypoglycaemia, cardiac troubles, urinary diseases, etc.

Though it is said that prevention is better than cure, the author is of the firm view that prevention is the only cure and that there is no cure apart from prevention. Once this truth is realised, one will take to natural hygiene (Nature cure) like a duck taking to water where no remedy is prescribed except to stress on the law of cause and effect.

Readers will benefit all the more by studying the companion volume "The Secrets of Wellness".

The author owes all what is stated herein to Sri Swami Pranava Brahmendra Ananda Saraswati, Paramahamsa Swami Sivananda Saraswati and Acharya Lakshmana Sarma. May the blessings of these holy personages be upon all readers, families and friends. By disseminating this sacred message among the public, the holy saints will shower their blessings all the time on all the followers. Let everyone thus offer his daily worship at the altar of Mother Nature.

S. Swaminathan

Natural Hygiene

asic Nature cure or natural hygiene is that branch of the science of life which deals with the care of the organism in a state of dis-ease or disease. It recognises that there is a law of health, which is also the law of cure and that by obedience to this law, health and healing are obtained. It includes all hygienic measures such as proper dieting, fasting, rest and relaxation, exercise (active, corrective and recreational), *pranayama*, sunbathing and hydrotherapy, which form part of the five-fold food medicine. There is no place in this science for drugs of any kind or for electrical, mechanical or other applications or so-called aids, which ultimately impair or endanger health. Non-violence to the human organism is accepted as the basic principle governing the application of Nature cure measures advocated herein.

Health Maxims

What is health?

- The human being is a triple unity of body, mind and spirit. Health depends upon caring for the body, caring for the mind and caring for the spirit as Nature intends the human being to care for them.

- Health is a positive state of well-being of the body, the mind and intellect (not just the absence of disease) — the health level of a person is to be assessed in the proper manner by finding out as to what extent the indicators of health are present in him.

- In the state of health there is evenness in the distribution of heat (known as body temperature) all over the body.

- A healthy person experiences a unique sense of lightness, not to be mistaken for weakness in the body, enabling him him to carry on the external and internal activities easily.

- In a state of health there is a feeling of comfort (*sukham*) all the time, with the feeling arising out of the body's internal cleanliness.

- Hunger is an indication of health; the keenness of hunger felt in a state of health enables the person to enjoy the taste of natural food. Good digestion would always be a part and parcel of it.

- A healthy person would be able to enjoy deep sleep for a few hours at night daily. On getting up from bed next morning, he feels fresh and full of energy.
- The bloodstream inside is clean and the skeletal and muscular systems are in tone. The healthy person will be able to discharge his daily duties very comfortably. He would not have any aversion to work.
- All his organs of excretion with none of them being overtaxed will discharge their functions satisfactorily, ensuring freedom from toxaemia from within.

The life power (*prana shakti*)

- What activates every cell/tissue within is the life power which is super physical and super chemical, not capable of being manufactured or obtained either from within or from outside through any activity.
- This life power is endowed on the infant at birth by Mother Nature. In other words, it is inherent in the organism.
- The life power so endowed in the infant is as it were kept as a reserve somewhere within known as *prana shakti*, but where the reserve is kept is unknown to man.
- To enable the body, the mind, etc. to carry on their internal and external functions day after day, a small quantum of power is released from the reserve. Such release takes place while one is asleep at night.
- The energy that is made available to the person on getting up from bed can be termed as vital power or *jeevan shakti*.
- There can be no action — physical or mental, external or internal, without a corresponding expenditure of power; the power so spent on every activity is that of *jeevan shakti*.
- In a body that is clean inside, the activities that go on are

termed as physiological activities. In a body that has become unclean, the activity of *jeevan shakti* (to eliminate the toxic matter from within) is called pathological activity.

- There is no dividing line between the physiological and pathological activities. In reality it is one continuous biological activity that goes on inside.

What is disease?

- The symptoms are not the disease. Suppressing the symptoms through the use of drugs (wrongly called medicines) is illogical, irrational and unhygienic.
- Behind all diseases, lies a cause which no drugs can reach.
- By adopting unhygienic habits of life quite an amount of *jeevan shakti* is wasted day after day; the eliminatory activities of the body suffer adversely and the body becomes unclean internally.
- Adoption of unhygienic activities results in enervation. Enervation leads to defective elimination, which results in accumulation of un-eliminated toxic matter (a state known as toxaemia). Toxaemia is the universal basic cause of disease right from the common cold to the much dreaded cancer and AIDS.
- *Jeevan shakti* does not keep any dirty matter within the body. When such matter accumulates over a period of time, *jeevan shakti* suspends most of the functions of the body and concentrates on eliminating the accumulated dirty matter. The person experiences symptoms like the common cold, cough, boils, loose motions, vomiting, etc. This is the acute stage of the disease.
- The disease is called acute when the *jeeven shakti* becomes vigorous (or acute). The term acute is not to be mistaken as 'serious'.
- Thus the passive cause of disease is the accumulated dirty matter within, while the active cause is the *jeevan shakti*.

- The vigorous elimination of unwanted foreign matter from within lasts only a short time. As a large part of available *jeevan shakti* is engaged in such an extraordinary elimination, the person concerned experiences weakness in his skeletal muscles, lack of hunger, coated tongue and inability to attend to normal intellectual activities.

- Such an acute form of disease is in reality intended to help the person to restore his internal sanitation back to normalcy.

- Where the symptoms of acute disease are sought to be suppressed through the use of drugs or in any other mechanical manner without employing any drugs, the internal uncleanliness of the body increases slowly and steadily leading to the onset of one or another type of chronic disease.

- Unlike the acute disease which lasts only two to four days at a time, chronic disease, e.g. asthma, bronchitis, high blood pressure, low blood pressure, heart trouble, joint diseases, sluggish liver, etc. is present for a fairly long time—for months, even years. In this state the daily availability of *jeevan shakti* depletes and the toxic matter inside steadily increases. Use of drugs and continued adoption of unhygienic living habits worsen the health level further.

- When the basic cause of chronic disease is not understood by the sufferer and when the symptoms are sought to be relieved by a drug or in any other mechanical manner disregarding the working of the law of cause and effect, the person concerned hops on to the third stage of disease termed as destructive disease, like epilepsy, TB, cancer, AIDS, etc.

- Disease in its primary stage is termed as acute disease; in its state of 'graduation', it turns chronic and the 'postgraduate' state of disease is destructive. Hence, wisdom lies in not allowing the progression of disease to occur in the body.

Prevention of disease

- All destructive diseases can be effectively prevented — and this is the only sane method of prevention — by not 'treating' chronic diseases the drug way or in any other mechanical manner. All chronic diseases can be prevented by not 'treating' acute disease irrationally through drugs, etc.

- As the state of disease implies some discomfort, minor or major, to the sufferer, the wise ones should not only learn to prevent chronic and destructive diseases but also practically apply such knowledge in day-to-day life. This is what the science of natural hygiene elaborates in detail.

- Any attempt to 'prevent' this or that disease through so-called inoculation, vaccination, etc. is but a futile effort for, only living hygienically can prevent disease. Health is the way; there is no way to health.

- Whenever a person takes a drug or vaccination or inoculation, etc., he only transplants the disease for future use.

- Let not the acute disease be suppressed. No chronic disease can develop in the person. The question of developing destructive disease will not at all arise.

- When a patient suffering from a chronic or destructive disease takes to the hygienic way of living and proceeds to rebuild his health the sane and safe way, the vital power or *jeevan shakti* in him as part of the internal cleansing process, brings on a healing crisis. Each such healing crisis (for a short period) is brought about for the specific purpose of raising the patient's health level.

- Since all disease implies tissue uncleanliness within, the cause of all disease is one. There are not many diseases, there is only one, i.e. lowered level of health. This principle is termed as the unity of disease.

- Disease can be radically cured by restoration of the health level of the patient by adopting the hygienic way of living. The cause of all disease being one, the treatment is also one, viz. restoration of health level back to normalcy by living in tune with the laws of health. This is known as unity of treatment.

- When there is but only a minor accumulation of toxaemia within and when *jeevan shakti* occasionally (say once in six or eight months) initiates a vigorous activity to eliminate it, such elimination occurs for improving the health of the body. This principle is known as the unity of health and disease.

- Even in the chronic and destructive stages of disease, when natural hygiene is followed, the life's 'will to health' asserts itself periodically through cleansing of the body by bringing on the healing crises.

- The principle of 'unity of cause' elucidates that the cause of all disease is one.

- The common notion prevalent in the society is that a diseased person has to take some medicine to cure his disease. The science of natural hygiene calls upon man to avoid the use of poisons (which all drugs are) and take to a sensible and limited intake of natural food during the diseased stage for radically curing the disease. This principle is termed as the 'unity of food and medicine'.

- What food is in a state of health and what as food can help to build up the health level of a person can alone serve as a medicine when a person falls ill. What is not food in health can never be medicine in disease.

- The body of a human being is made up of five elements of Nature, viz. *akash* (ether), air, natural light (*agni*), water and earth (meaning the edible plant foods growing out of earth).

- Each of these five elements is food for man. Thus food is five-fold. Any deficiency in the supply of any of these elements will result in internal imbalance or ill health.

- As the principle of unity of food and medicine operates all through, only these five elements can serve as man's medicines. This principle is known as the five-fold food medicine.

- All chemicals, all metallic products and every kind of poison extracted from the bodies of animals, reptiles, etc. can never be medicine for man.

- As Dr Henry Lindlahr has effectively put it: "All the *materia medica* as at present known were to be sunk to the bottom of the sea, it will be all the better for mankind and all the worse for fishes."

- In place of *materia medica* available in the different systems of medication, natural hygiene advocates the adoption of *materia hygienica* as a positive aid to health. Poisons and non-food products can never serve the purpose of nectar. Let Nature be the guide and let her dictates be followed scrupulously.

- Some micro-organisms (germs, bacilli, microbes, etc.) may be seen in the pathogenic matter but to mistake the germs as the cause of disease is totally wrong.

- In many disease conditions, germ activity may be there. Killing the germs concerned through drugs, etc. may give temporary symptomatic relief, but the fact is that the health level never improves. It goes on steadily worsening instead.

- Natural hygiene clearly proves that germs are not the cause of disease. If the germ theory were true, no disease can be cured through adoption of natural hygiene for in this system, we never employ any germ-killing measures. The fact is that even medical failures are radically cured through the adoption of natural hygiene.

- If the germ theory were true, there would be no disease without the so-called causative germs clearly visible inside. The fact is that in so many disease conditions the so-called causative germs are not visible when the disease is in its early stages.

- The germ is but a *bhangi* (cleaner, scavenger) recruited by Mother Nature for clearing the dirt from within. As George Bernard Shaw, famous playwright, has put it: "These human beings are suffering from horrible diseases, they infect us poor microbes and you doctors pretend that it is we who infect them."

- It is plainly admitted by bacteriologists that the so-called medicines administered for killing germs really add to the resistance power of the germs. The germs subjected to such torture become drug resistant. A stage is reached when no drug whatever can ever 'control' the symptoms of the disease.

- Let not suppression of symptoms through drugs be adopted.

- Chronic and destructive diseases will be totally rid of if we do not kill the *bhangi* or the scavenger who has entered at the behest of Mother Nature to cleanse the body from within.

Food and energy

- The prevalent notion mistakenly taken as scientific that food is the source of energy is the reason why numerous persons eat without hunger, or eat even when they clearly know that they cannot digest the food taken by them.

- The intake of food by a person may create a psychological feeling that 'he has supplied energy to the body', and it may make him temporarily feel better even though no physiological benefit is derived.

- What activates every cell and tissue within the organism is the *jeevan shakti*, which cannot be produced by the food taken inside the body. Digestion of food is a vital action necessitating the expenditure of *jeevan shakti* (vital power). It is unscientific to hold that an activity, which involves expenditure of power, supplies power to the body.

- As Acharya Lakshmana Sarma, who is hailed as father of Nature cure, has practically proved that food is a tax on vitality; common sense decrees that there should be the minimum of tax imposed on vitality, i.e. just to the extent needed and no more.

- Where the food eaten is natural and is digested properly, the body gets therefrom the requisite blood sugar, amino acids, the needed fatty acids, different types of vitamins and mineral salts, enzymes, trace elements, water and the cellulose or roughage, required for keeping the body chemistry in order. All these are 'matter' and not energy.

- When the requisite vitamins, etc. are supplied to the body in the natural form, the body is able to keep the structure of the different organs in proper shape. In that ideal condition, *jeevan shakti*, manifests itself through the different organs, i.e. with the least expenditure of *jeevan shakti*. Where the wrong type of food is supplied and where many of these natural nutrients are not available to the body inside, the concerned structures become weak and the person concerned feels weak.

- Thus food is not a source of energy; it is a medium through which energy is expressed.

Healthy dietetics

- Eat only when hungry and that too moderately (i.e. not more than half the stomach load at any given time and not more than twice a day).

- The load on the digestive system becomes unbearable if a person eats three or four times a day.

- Work and digestion do not go together. When there is work, keep the stomach as little loaded as possible. At this stage take only raw vegetables, seasonal fruits or their juices.

- Take the main meal at the end of the day when all work is over and then go to sleep comfortably without the world disturbing you. Even the night meal has to be moderate in quantity.

- Keep away from all bottled foods, tinned foods, manufactured and preserved foods, etc. Take only natural foods—food items as provided to human kind by Nature.

- Refining of cereals robs the foodgrains of many nutrients like vitamins, minerals, etc. As Sir William Arbuthnot Lane has put it: "The whiter the bread the sooner you are dead."

- Whatever could be consumed raw, uncooked, let that be taken in its original form. Whatever needs cooking let it be steamed. Let it be cooked in the steam cooker. Overcooking, frying, etc. should be avoided.

- Fruits ripened artificially through chemicals, cold storage — i.e. not being fresh — are unfit for human health. Milk should be fresh; the longer the milk is kept on the shelves the more useless it becomes. Pasteurised milk is stale milk.

- Where fresh milk is not available, one can remind oneself that none other than human beings consume the milk of other animals. It is possible to live healthy without milk and milk products. Thousands of vegetarians are living in different parts of the globe without meat and fish. If the vegetarian diet is properly planned, one can live without milk or milk products too.

- The body requires a moderate supply of predominantly alkaline foods day after day. Such foods are vegetables, fruits, etc. that should predominate in the diet and be supplemented by a small quantity of unrefined cereals, etc.

- Predominantly acidic foods such as refined cereals, de-husked pulses and grams, refined flour, white sugar, stale milk, flesh foods, eggs, confectionery and hydrogenated oils have a deleterious impact on human health.

Vital economy and non-violence

- As *jeevan shakti* is wasted when one adopts unhygienic activities, common sense decrees that only hygienic habits be adopted in daily life. These have to be adopted in tune with the principle of vital economy and non-violence to produce the best results.
- The principle of vital economy — a principle which finds mention only in the science of natural hygiene — implies that only such actions should be done by the human being that result in the least possible expenditure of *jeevan shakti*.
- Sticking to the principle of non-violence in daily life ensures the correct observance of the principle of vital economy.

Fasting

- Periodical fasting even when one is healthy ensures the observance of vital economy.
- The daily programme of living has to be so designed that no organ in the body is over-worked, that no organ is (through the use of drugs or mechanical, electrical or other contrivances) forced to function in a particular manner, that basic needs of life are supplied in the right and balanced proportion as it is essential to ensure that no violence whatever is inflicted on any organ inside. Every act of violence enervates the organism and the health-seeker has to acquire the requisite knowledge as to what results and what does not result in such violence.

- Fast of a short duration of one or two days may be undertaken even when one is healthy.
- In acute diseases, total fasting would help in radically curing the disease quickly. In chronic diseases partial fasting is to be resorted to by the concerned patient. In destructive diseases the approach to fasting is to be resorted to and when conditions improve positively, partial fasting may be undertaken.
- Fasting is not starvation. The fear that fasting can weaken the body is baseless.
- As and when there are healing crises, treat them on par with acute disease and fast accordingly.
- Every health-promoting application like non-violent *pranayama*, the spinal bath, the non-violent enema, etc. have to be resorted to well within the limits imposed by the principles of vital economy and non-violence. If this is borne in mind, the best possible results will follow.
- Attempting to get symptomatic relief from distressing symptoms through the use of mechanical or electrical contrivances may seem drugless cures but the relief obtained is in violation of the law of cause and effect. These methods/applications should not find place in the programme of one who has taken to natural hygiene. Natural hygiene has enough practical guidance to give to the sufferer to enable him to obtain the much needed symptomatic relief.

Mental health

- A calm mind hastens recovery from disease, as it ensures that the glands and nerves in the organism work far better.
- The very adoption of a disciplined way of life as advocated by natural hygiene helps in controlling the mind sensibly and the sense organs properly.

- The discipline involved will calm down the mind and improve the power of intellect considerably.
- Adoption of natural hygiene in daily life combined with daily prayers to Almighty and proper attention to cultivation of virtues like humility, sincerity, magnanimity, etc. would go a long way in enabling man to move on the path towards perfection.
- What is needed is understanding and sincere application of the principles involved.
- While every hygienic habit is welcome, it is unwise to choose one such habit alone and to follow it to the exclusion of various other hygienic habits as it would be purposeless. Let the 'total approach' be adopted by every health-seeker.

Maintenance of Body Ecology

Efforts to restore normal environment

Everyone is aware of the fact that since about A.D. 1930 the modern world has been facing various ecological problems, which are affecting the progress of mankind in every field. Sincere and serious efforts are being made at various levels the world over to deal with these issues effectively.

Even the common man is aware of the problems posed by air, water and noise pollution. The havoc wrought by these types of pollution on human health is but common knowledge. Authorities at various levels — governmental and non-governmental — are anxious to mitigate, if not totally eliminate, these types of pollution. Destruction and denudation of forests have a serious adverse effect on the overall economic development of the world. Hence, afforestation is being resorted to.

Even in the field of destruction of wildlife which again has a serious impact on the maintenance of ecology of the world, efforts are on to see that such destructive efforts are totally prohibited.

Raising the human health level

All these laudable efforts are being undertaken for the benefit of future generations of mankind. Is the same attention being paid for improving the physical and mental health of man? If the answer to

1

this question is in the affirmative we will be happy for ecological improvement with diseased men in society would be a meaningless proposition.

Is it not then our duty to see to it that with constructive efforts for ecological improvement of the world, productive steps in the not far off future are taken for creating a disease-free society? Let us aim at a world wherein all its inhabitants would enjoy good physical and mental health, each co-operating with the other and, if I am not a dreamer, to see that utopia becomes a reality on this planet. Let us investigate the matter further.

Focus on the vital problem

The family is the unit of society. Unless and until each member of the family becomes health conscious, unless and until he/she is enabled to live healthy, disease-free in tune with eternal, immutable and inviolable laws of life, mere ecological development on proper lines may not improve the general health level of humanity.

Whether one likes it or not, the world today is full of diseases. No doubt efforts are on to keep diseases under control, but health in the real sense of the term is becoming more and more a rarity in modern civilisation. Why? Let us probe further.

The present tendency in society the world over is to consider that the incidence of disease in human beings is inevitable, that the different diseases are brought to mankind by viruses, germs, bacilli, microbes and the like, that admittedly there are many incurable, chronic and destructive diseases to which persons succumb at middle age, that there is apparently no way to make the entire mankind free from such chronic and destructive diseases. To sum up, there is all around a hopeless attitude of pessimism — whatever high sounding technical jargons are mouthed by 'experts' and whatever 'breakthroughs' are 'advertised' through the media by the drugs industry from time to time.

The solution out of this miserable state lies somewhere else. It lies in a sphere which neither an expert nor an industry seems to probe into and here is the right royal road to health.

Health is man's birthright. The human mechanism is so designed that it can carry on all the activities inside very effectively. The mechanism is perfect. All that is needed is for the modern man to recognise the truth, understand it fully and start living in tune with the laws of life. Thus alone can the body ecology be kept up and the right maintenance of body ecology is health.

Man's efforts for re-establishment of health have been proceeding on wrong lines for quite some decades. It is a pity that more often than not the symptoms are mistaken for disease, that symptomatic relief through the employment of poisonous drugs is hailed as the cure of disease and, where a disease is admitted even by medicos to be an incurable one, to keep a semblance of normalcy regular use of drugs is made as an effort to keep the disease under control.

Nowhere is the truth normally recognised that a disease can be radically cured only by removing the fundamental cause of the disease, i.e. unhygienic living. Nowhere is the truth perceived that disease in reality is a diminution in the level of health brought about by unhygienic living. Nowhere it is realised that the cure lies in the removal of the cause of disease.

Nature cure approach

In this perverse atmosphere we plead for return to sanity. As we happen to be numerically in a minority, our voice is dismissed. When we say that the germs are not the real cause of disease, our case is not heard. Such is the adamant attitude of the majority.

3

If Nature cure is becoming more and more popular, it is because the hopelessly incurable cases are more in despair, turning towards the system of thought which firmly holds that Nature and Nature alone could heal.

Let us at least now take a U-turn and start on the path of health. Enough groundwork has already been done in this regard by Louis Kuhne, Revered Father Kneipp, Dr Henry Lindlahr, Dr John H. Tilden, Dr R.T. Trall, Dr Herbert M. Shelton, Dr Stanley Lief and Acharya Lakshmana Sarma and several others. They have explained how and why disease is caused, how health can be restored by simple natural methods by having nothing to do with chemicals or non-plant products.

What these personages have elaborated can be summed up in a *sutra* form in just one sentence of Acharya Lakshmana Sarma: "*Health is the way; there is no way to health.*"

Acharya Lakshmana Sarma pleaded with the modern individual to restore his/her body ecology. The body ecology cannot be maintained properly and the person cannot be healthy in the real sense of the term

- unless and until the structural integrity of each organ inside the human body is maintained well;
- unless and until the life force or *prana shakti* inside the human organism is, without being wasted in any way, allowed to flow through the nervous system, enabling each organ to maintain its functional efficiency;
- unless and until the production of waste matter within the human body is kept within sensible limits;
- unless and until the eliminatory organs are allowed to clear the internal dirty matter;
- unless and until adequate rest — physical, sensory, emotional and physiological — is made available to the indi-

vidual. The health *sutra*, therefore, boils down to: "Be conscious about body ecology and maintain it."

The science of natural hygiene is one which is based on the eternal, inviolable and immutable laws of life. By living in tune with these laws, the ill can become well, the well can become better and the better can become still better.

Laws of life

The laws of life are Nature's laws (not man-made) which state that:

- The primal energy behind the systematic, orderly and continued working of the different organs all through life — known as 'life power' or *prana shakti* is superphysical, super chemical — are not the 'product' of any bodily activity or of any external material influence.

- The vital power is not to be wasted or squandered away in fruitless or unhygienic living as such wasteful effort would bring on disease, debility, etc.

- Hygienic living alone can contribute to a progressive improvement in health.

- Where due to the adoption of some unhygienic habits the body has become internally insanitary, the 'vital power', assuming the role of 'healing power', starts vigorous elimination through the process of acute disease for restoring internal sanitation, that is, normalcy in health.

- No suppressive measures should be adopted for obtaining symptomatic relief; adopting hygienic measures aimed at restoration of blood purity, better blood circulation, etc. are the only way out.

- Mental states such as inferiority complex, depression, etc., that is, the emotional upsets leading to development of

5

anger, jealousy and the like can cause serious harm to the health of nervous and glandular systems. Based upon the perception of this truth the human being should make positive and constructive efforts to restore calmness and composure of mind.

The basic needs of the body — food, water, air, exercise (hygienic, educational and corrective), rest, relaxation, sleep, etc. and the basic mental needs like integrity, character, happiness, contentment, etc. should be made available to the body and mind in proper proportions to enable the organism to work in the right direction.

This brief narration of the laws of life is only meant as a guidance. It is only when the science of Nature cure is studied in depth and practised in daily life that the truth behind the laws can be perceived fully.

During the past two centuries thousands of chronically ill the world over have radically recovered from chronic ailments like asthma, bronchitis, blood pressure, heart disease, tumours, cancer, etc.

The primitive man instinctively knew this secret. As civilisation started progressing and as persons became addicted to unnatural habits and customs, the knowledge of this natural science was ignored. This was the original *Ayurveda* system involving no type of medication except a sensible diet, fasting, better breathing and manageable physical activities.

My experience of over five decades has convinced me of the utility of this science for all, for the unhealthy as well as for the healthy persons. By following the principles enunciated in this science, the body ecology can be restored and once this ecology is restored to a normal or near normal condition, diseases would take 'French leave'.

Indicators of health

Health is a positive condition or state of the mind and body as indicated by:

- an even distribution of bodily heat (temperature) from head to foot;
- the feeling of lightness (freedom from any sense of heaviness anywhere in the body);
- experiencing a rare sense of comfort inside the body;
- keen hunger;
- ability to get sound sleep daily;
- ability in the muscles of the body to do the needed physical and mental or intellectual work;
- the capacity to do work without any aversion to doing it;
- the capacity in the eliminatory organs — the lungs, the kidneys, the bowels and skin to discharge their eliminatory activities without any strain, easily and comfortably;
- the experiencing of a sense of comfort (termed as *sukhanubhav*).

A really healthy person must be able to experience the cumulative effect of all the above features.

Nature cure: A way of life

Having stated what health is, let me reiterate that health is not mere absence of disease symptoms or discomfort. The science of Nature cure, the practice of which enables the individual to maintain his body ecology ideally or in a near ideal state is the only sane, safe and sensible method to keep oneself healthy and protect oneself from the clutches of diseases like blood pressure, heart diseases, cancer, etc. It is not just a system of therapeutics. It expounds a philosophy of life which, if understood or adopted by the healthy to keep themselves healthy all the time, would enable them to

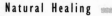

improve their health progressively and if adopted by the unhealthy, it can radically cure their so-called disease conditions.

Understanding the Precepts

Symbiosis

The human body is a community of organs. Each organ while discharging its function(s) also takes care of the welfare of the whole body, in many cases working as a 'partner' to one or more organs elsewhere in the body. The body structure when studied scientifically produces awe and wonder in our minds. There is as it were a perfect organisation working in tune with the laws of life and given the requisite hygienic care, every person can maintain his body ecology ideally.

It is the symbiotic relationship among the various organs of the body that ensures that all physiological actions inside take place with a purpose. Even the so-called pathological activity is set ultimately to restore the normal balance within, if only man does not interfere or suppress or complicate the internal condition. He ought to have the common sense to understand that he has no alternative but to follow the dictates of Mother Nature and restore normalcy within before disorder (which has caused the pathological action) worsens beyond the tolerable extent.

The organisation within

The arrangement of various organs inside the human body, the manner in which each organ discharges its function(s) effectively—

so effectively that the human being is not even aware of anything that is going on inside — the quickness with which new cells are manufactured all twenty-four hours of the day and the manner in which old cells are being replaced; the almost incomprehensible arrangement as to how even while the heart and the lungs work non-stop, they are taking the much needed rest every day; the manner in which the tiny zygote formed at the time of conception grows systematically and methodically into a human babe in nine months and a few odd days; the ease with which, in a perfect state of health the woman is able to deliver a full-grown babe; the arrangement which makes it possible for the female breast to produce milk (giving the needed nutrition) for the baby; the fine system which regulates the baby's physical and mental growth through the years of childhood and adolescence — all these indicate that there is an 'order' within the human organism. And this order is there in every living being the entire world over. Should not common sense suggest that if there is to be such order prevalent the world over, if there is such an order inside each human being, there should be an Ordainer behind that order? Can there be an order alone without an Ordainer behind co-ordinating, regulating, directing and ensuring that the order is kept up all the time?

Somatic awareness

In maintaining the organisation each cell in the body plays its role in the manner designed by Nature. Each living cell is endowed with an instinct of self-preservation. It is this instinct that makes it possible for every cell to know what nutrients it must take in from the general bloodstream and what waste materials it must eliminate in order to keep itself clean and healthy. This awareness in each living cell is termed 'somatic awareness'. The presence of somatic awareness in each cell is part of the order referred to above.

Now let us direct our attention as to who the Ordainer is because an understanding of this vital piece of knowledge is very essential for keeping the body free from chronic and destructive diseases, that is, in other words keeping the body healthy all through life.

That Ordainer is there in each human being. It is 'power'. It is energy, totally different from the power (the energy) that we human beings produce through mechanical means in the world. The vital energy within the human organism and the mechanical energy produced by man in the world are totally different: one is not interchangeable with the other.

After all we have to express our ideas through words. If some words can fit in for that, that Ordainer is life power or *prana shakti* or *prana*. If this *prana* is not there in the human body — and this is what the term death connotes — disorganisation sets in and disintegration goes on unchecked.

The human body may look like a machine. It is possible to describe the manner of working of each organ in mechanical terms. Let it be understood that through chemicals and poisons man can stimulate (or irritate) the working of the organs. He can employ sedatives or tranquillisers (these are really chemical substances) to 'calm one organ or the other'. He can transplant the kidney or the heart or some other organ. He can delude himself that he has 'normalised the internal functions', but let it be remembered that these are only forced actions, forced on the system. No one can annul the internal arrangement. If an organ is forced to work in a particular direction, the body would suffer adversely. Such forced action results from extraordinary expenditure of the vital power within.

Let it be realised that every so-called mechanical aid (it could be chemical or non-chemical) used from outside is a *prana*-waster.

As this *prana* cannot be had from any source whatever from outside or from inside the human body, the individual who wastes his *prana* in the manner indicated does it at the risk of losing his health by stages.

Prana is the Ordainer behind the order within. Wisdom decrees that this power should not be wasted. What this *prana* is, is a mystery to all except the few gifted individuals who have advanced on the spiritual path through practical spiritual *sadhana*.

Constitution

Though the age of the human being is counted from the date of his birth on Earth, the *prana* in that individual starts working from the time the conception took place. *Prana* keeps itself busy during the intra-uterine period in building up the body structure of the baby and this process generally takes a period of nine months and a few odd days when the baby is delivered.

The physical frame endowed on the baby (by the mother) at the time of its birth could be termed as constitution. The sounder the constitution of a baby the more long-lived and healthy the person will be. Conversely the weaker the constitution the less healthy the person will be. He will also be short-lived.

Pregnancy is not a disease. It does not require any medical care. If during pregnancy a mother is sensible enough to supply what the foetus needs for building up its constitution, if she takes the proper pre-natal care to keep her system, especially the strength of her pelvic musculature, healthy, childbirth cannot present any difficulty whatsoever.

A weak constitution cannot be strengthened to any extent, by any effort made after the child's birth. But a sound constitution can be weakened and weakened slowly and steadily by improper infant care, improper child care, bad psychological handling of the child and adolescent by the mother/father/teacher. Each of these contributes to the health of the adult to be. Each of these has a social obligation towards mankind. All through life, hygienic care has to be taken by each person so that the constitution is not weakened. The structure of the human body is so designed that as years advance, it goes on depreciating, though very slowly, almost imperceptibly. However living in tune with the laws of life will ensure that a fairly good level of health is maintained even in old age. Old age need neither be senility nor disability nor deformity.

Premature ageing and the development of chronic and destructive diseases are the consequences of erratic living, which is what is loosely known as the civilised way of life. I am not for a moment calling upon people to be uncivilised. But my plea is, 'Be civilised without suffering.' Such habits as are mistaken to be civilised ways of life but which are unhealthy and unhygienic, ought to be given the go by. The reason why so many diseases are rampant in the present world is because man is not primarily health conscious and he is influenced by advertisers and commercial interests.

Be prudent. Prudence calls on every human being to live long and live healthy.

If all the care and attention is taken by a person the integrity of structure of every organ will be ideal or near ideal all through life. The functional efficiency of each organ would also be in a similar state. The human being has to keep up the structural integrity and functional efficiency of the organs within, all through his life by ensuring that his daily habits are in tune with the laws of life. If this care is slackened or lost, both functional efficiency and structural integrity suffer and the body ecology is not maintained.

Nature cure is essentially Nature care. The human being is a triple unity of body, mind and spirit. Acharya Lakshmana Sarma says, *"Care for your body, care for your mind and care for your spirit as Nature intends you to care for them."* There is no alternative to this.

Structural Integrity and Functional Efficiency

Structural integrity

Each organ and each tissue is composed of cells. The cell is the unit of structure. Each cell positioned at its appropriate place is guided by the life power or *prana shakti* within and thus each living cell has the requisite functional power in it. Each of these cells, wherever it may be located, has two fundamental functions:

- Nutrition, i.e. the power to assimilate its nutritional requirements through the bloodstream.
- Drainage, i.e. the ability to remove the unwanted waste matter through the different eliminatory organs in the body.

Each cell has an instinctive awareness termed as somatic awareness, which enables it to be aware of what its functions are, what nutrients it must take in from blood for maintaining its health and what it should eliminate in order to keep itself clean and healthy.

In an ideal state of health, somatic awareness of each cell is present to the appropriate extent. It is only when the body becomes enervated due to the concerned person living unhygienically and when for a period of time proper nutrients are not supplied to the organism through the general bloodstream, that somatic awareness of the cells starts going down by stages.

When somatic awareness dicreases, the different organs in the body start faltering in their functions, the tissues inside become unclean, the eliminatory organs fail to discharge their duties and man becomes diseased.

It is but logical to conclude that any amount of drug treatment cannot normalise the functions within or restore somatic awareness of the cells. Proper maintenance of body ecology and proper maintenance of health of each cell depends upon only one factor, viz. living in tune with the laws of life.

Functional efficiency

Only when each system has the requisite functional efficiency to discharge its functions fully as designed by Nature can one be healthy. No organ, no tissue inside the body is unimportant and every organ, every tissue must have its functional efficiency. Functional efficiency depends upon the following:

- Adequate supply of nerve energy to each cell. Such supply can be ensured only through observance of the principles of vital economy.
- Supply of the basic needs of living, i.e. air, water, food, exercise, rest or repose to the body, day after day. If any basic need is over-supplied or if any basic need is denied even to some extent, one or more organ inside may develop derangement of functions leading to a fall in the functional efficiency of different systems.
- Proper maintenance of posture while sitting, standing, working, walking and sleeping.
- Proper maintenance of emotional poise while attending to the day's activities, as lack of emotional poise affects the glandular and nervous systems in the body leading to loss of functional efficiency in one or more systems.

- No non-food product, chemical or any inorganic sub-stance, is to be shoved into the body. Such products, as not part of the basic needs of living, would cause the vital power or *jeevan shakti* to direct itself in doing unwanted activities.

- Strict adherence to the adoption of the principle of non-violence guides in planning one's programme of daily life.

- Non-use of electrical or mechanical appliances or mea-sures like violent massage, ostensibly to 'normalise' one internal function or the other (which might have earlier become abnormal).

- Fasting to the extent required as and when needed.

- Taking in of predominantly positive food to the extent needed and in the manner indicated in the science of natural hygiene.

- Observance of sensible control over the working of the ten sense organs in the body. Five of them are known as or-gans of perception or *jnanendriyas*, i.e. the skin, the eyes, the ears, the tongue (as organ of taste) and the nose. Five of them are known as organs of action or *karmendriyas*, i.e. the tongue (as the organ of speech), the hands, the feet, the anus and the reproductory organ.

- Activity — proper physiological functioning of the differ-ent organs, performance of one's external (worldly) activi-ties, exercise just to the extent needed — has to be a part of the daily routine.

The different systems can be functionally efficient only if the structure of each organ is proper in the manner designed by Nature. Special attention must be paid to maintenance of structural integrity of vital organs like the brain, the lungs, the heart, the liver, the kidneys, etc. Any derangement in the structure of any of these vital organs is bound to adversely and seriously affect the body's functioning as a whole. Thus, the subject of structural integrity assumes a vital importance in the proper maintenance of body ecology.

For maintenance of structural integrity, the person concerned should so fashion his daily programme of living that he does not develop any obesity or emaciation. In both these cases the body starts accumulating within it encumberances, leading to loss of structural integrity of one organ or the other and loss of functional efficiency too.

If functional efficiency is properly maintained and the daily programme of living is on hygienic lines, structural integrity of each organ would be maintained properly. No additional precautions are needed.

While the ideal has been set out above, the writer admits that modern social conditions create a situation wherein the practice of one or the other ideals appears difficult. Care should be taken to see that such lapses are not frequent. Where as a result of occasional lapse(s) a slight derangement of this or that function within is felt by a person, let him take due note of it as early as possible. He should set things right through the practical applications advocated in the science of natural hygiene, such as the cooling abdominal wet pack, the spinal bath, the non-violent enema, the 'tickling' massage, approach to fasting, etc. Let every slight abnormality within become normal in the strict non-violent way and in tune with the principle of vital economy. Let no person 'force' normalcy through any unnatural method. It is the repeated resort to such 'forceful' methods that leads one to chronic and destructive diseases wherein the structural integrity of one or more vital organ is adversely affected. Hence, let due care be exercised through the sensible practical applications of natural hygiene to normalise the system at an early stage.

The science of natural hygiene is one which helps the ill to become well, the well to become better and the better to become still better. Let not this system be considered as an alternative system of medicine as many people take it to be. Though this is not a system of therapeutics, the term 'Nature cure' has stuck to it. Let every reader study natural hygiene in depth and practise it all through life. Illness can be avoided, health of body and mind can be maintained and, above all, natural happiness can be experienced throughout life.

Cleanliness

A basic need

Around the middle of the 19th century Rev. Father Sebastian Kneipp, a Nature cure pioneer, said, "*All disease is but tissue uncleanliness.*"

This sums up the problem very aptly. Only when the tissues inside the body are rendered unclean that there is disease in the body. What Dr John H. Tilden, another of our pioneers, referred to as toxaemia being the sole cause of all disease in the body is identical to what Sebastian Kneipp had said.

It is man's unhygienic way of living that makes his body internally unclean, diseased. When man enervates himself through adoption of unhealthy habits of living, his eliminatory organs cannot clear the entire dirt from within as his *jeevan shakti* is wrongly spent on many useless activities, physical and mental.

How then can man achieve the requisite standard of cleanliness or can he set right his body ecology? The answer is to divert the *jeeven shakti* to remove the offending matter from within and re-establish internal sanitation. This is what the science of natural hygiene elaborates upon.

In the world outside everything is sought to be kept clean. External sanitation is sought to be maintained through all possible efforts, thanks to town planning and sustained efforts of engineers and sanitation experts. Every place is sought to look as clean as possible.

Let us study the situation that prevailed long ago. Though located in the temperate zone, Great Britain witnessed the epidemic of smallpox once every four or five year regularly in the 18th and 19th centuries. The government compulsorily foisted on every citizen, including the adult citizens, compulsory vaccination, and revaccination against smallpox once every five years. In spite of repeated vaccination, the incidence of smallpox rose regularly. The situation became intolerable. A few well-intentioned medical doctors in that country wondered whether vaccination was really the solution to the problem. They formed an Anti-Vaccination League of Great Britain and with the co-operation of other eminent citizens began to study the problem in depth. Towards the fag end of the 19th century, the County Council of Leicestershire took a decision that the entire money spent till then on vaccination should be diverted to improving external sanitation. When this decision was taken everyone in England forecast that most of the people of that county would die of smallpox before long. The other parts of the country went on with the vaccination campaign as before.

Leicestershire persisted in its sanitation campaign and won its battle, while the epidemic of smallpox raged in the rest of the country. The Leicestershire experiment 'enthused' the anti-vaccination league of Great Britain, which compelled the government to appoint a Royal Commission on Vaccination. This Royal Commission constituted in 1889 went into the whole question in depth. A minority of the members recorded a note of dissent and the Commission itself recommended the insertion of a conscience clause in the country's vaccination laws. This was about the beginning of the 20th century. Many citizens availed of the benefits of refusing vaccination. The number of persons refusing vaccination began to increase steadily year after year, correspondingly the incident of smallpox decreased and the British vaccination law was repealed in 1947.

When India became a republic in 1950, a number of medical experts from Great Britain submitted a petition to the Parliament of India to repeal the vaccination laws in India and free India from smallpox for ever. The petition, however, went unheard.

When the objective in England was achieved, the anti-vaccination league in that country was dissolved. The history concerning the activities of the National Anti-Vaccination League of Great Britain is present, as also is the report of the British Royal Commission on Vaccination for anyone to peruse. A brief narration of all these is given in Acharya Lakshmana Sarma's *Practical Nature Cure*.

Anyone that cares to study these facts will find that it was not vaccination but improvement in the external sanitation that achieved the miracle in Great Britain.

Let it be noted that all types of vaccination and inoculation are but filth-medication, not capable of eradicating any disease whatever. Acharya Lakshmana Sarma has called the vaccination method as filth-medication. Mahatma Gandhi was opposed to all types of vaccination. Doctor Creighton, one of the most eminent medical authorities of Great Britain, was requested in 1888 to write an article on vaccination for publication in the *Encyclopaedia Britannica*. Dr Creighton's article was a total condemnation of the system of vaccination. Though it was published in just one edition of the *Encyclopaedia*, it was left out in its later editions for reasons best known to the publishers of that encyclopaedia.

In fact, all the twenty-four doctors who submitted their petition to the Parliament of India in 1950, also condemned the practice of vaccination.

Thus, the only sensible solution to the problem of eradication of disease is to restore body ecology back to normalcy through adoption of hygienic living in tune with the laws of Nature.

The pollution problem

Lip sympathy is being paid to external sanitation. Everything may look glossy and clean, however, there can be no cleanliness worth its name so long as air pollution, water pollution, soil pollution (using artificial fertilisers), crop pollution (through the spray of insecticides and pesticides on crops), etc. continue. The bloodstream inside the body is getting more and more polluted by every one of these types of pollution.

Maybe, some of the industries that were established decades ago may have to be radically reconditioned or even 'liquidated'. However, in the interest of human health this apparently unpleasant step has to be taken by all interests concerned for advancement of human health. Let no one forget that unalterable fact that cleanliness within the human body can be maintained at a near ideal level only by ensuring that every human being gets clean water (unchlorinated, unfluoridated), clean air and clean surroundings. However, there is one more vital factor to be borne in mind by health-seekers, and that is mental cleanliness.

Man is a triple unity of body, mind, and spirit and man's fundamental duty is to care for his body, his mind and his spirit as Nature intends him to. Care of these cannot be taken unless and until every person is educated on the right lines to enable him to acquire emotional poise.

The fact is that the requisite level of emotional poise means a person should have the knowledge to deal with emotional conflicts that arise ordinarily. Through such mental conflicts, the glandular and nervous systems of the person get shattered, and the body ecology cannot be kept up or health be enjoyed.

In ordinary day-to-day life one faces complex situations or may have to work in unfavourable surroundings, where a basic knowledge of mind management (including time management) is to form a part of one's education at various levels. Having learnt the art of mind management, the person can go through such situations unruffled, unscathed and keep his body ecology in proper condition.

Clarity of Mind

In the last chapter the subject of cleanliness was dealt with as a pre-requisite to health, that is, cleanliness at the physical level (inwardly and outwardly). The topic here is the cleanliness at the mental level, i.e. clarity of mind.

The lowest order of creation, insects, worms, etc. are endowed with the instinct that guides them in all their activities. Even in the slightly higher order of creation, it is mostly the instinct that guides them in their day-to-day routine activities and even in ordinary circumstances. Instinct in these lower orders of creation is unperverted, i.e. as Nature has endowed them with. No outward influence has been exercised upon them to pervert their instincts.

Where man interferes with the natural life and habitat of animals (e.g. animals made use of to conduct scientific investigations or those 'trained' for circus purposes), the instincts naturally get perverted.

In what are known as scientific experiments on animals, pigs, rats, rabbits, monkeys and the like, experimenters have tried to condition their instincts to serve the purpose of experiment on hand. For instance, in a particular experiment numerous rats were being fed with a particular type of food. When the feeding was about to begin, a bell was rung. So the rats associated the ringing of bell to feeding time. After some days when the bell was rung, the rats rushed in for food, though they were not hungry as they had been fed only half an hour earlier. It looked at if the rats were ready for eating. Such experiments on animals, which in their wild state had unperverted instincts in them, could be conditioned to suit the whims of man, the so-called experimenter.

As for man himself there are ever so many influences in the modern world, each one being exerted by a category of persons with some specific interests in view. Even the basic instincts appear, more or less, to be perverted the entire world over. Education at various levels appears to be conditioning the mind of man so much that it is difficult to spot a human being today who would look at a problem completely unaffected or uninfluenced by the conditions or circumstances around him. Such a rare person who could bring about an originality in approach may be here or there in this wide world, but if such people exist, their example goes unnoticed, unsung and unrecognised.

Am I presenting a dismal picture of the state of affairs of the modern world? It is claimed that science and technology are raging ahead at full speed, that information technology is expanding, that a machine designed today for collating, analysing and storing scientific data becomes out-of-date the next month itself. Space research is proceeding at such a fast rate that man has started planning on how he can establish his habitation in the planets far, far away.

With such an impressive picture of scientific progress before mankind today, let us look at the other side. Man essentially lives on this planet for a few years. After the years of infancy he gets educated slowly and steadily, qualifies himself in some manner and on reaching adulthood he has 'to face the problems of livelihood'. All these require a basic ingredient — the original mind with clarity. One should be capable of understanding worldly knowledge imparted to him by different educational systems, of analysing the data collected by him, of using his own power of discrimination to sort out the grain from the chaff. He should be capable of endowing himself with the needed strength to face the problems of livelihood and the problems of life.

A major question before mankind today is: "Is enough attention being paid to enable man to develop his mind on the right lines with all the capabilities referred to in the preceding paragraph?" With everything in the modern world having been professionalised, each man today is utterly dependent upon this or that profession 'to solve' his problems, whatever these may be. There ought to be no great danger in such an arrangement if all people were selfless, without any kind of vested interest. Such professionals without professionalism, unfortunately, are very rare in this world. And the common man gets exploited by either this or that professional. The fact is that one professional exploits the other professional. Such exploitation is among those engaged in scientific research while in the moral or ethical sense, there ought not to be such competition among such persons.

With this 'exploitation unlimited' having become universal, no one seems to be happy in the modern world. On the one hand, information on knowledge is accumulating day after day while on the other, almost every man is plagued by emotional conflicts. Quite a few are so tense that they 'need' tranquillisers and sedatives.

Is this state of affairs a happy one? Is not the basic requirement of man a capability to sort out his own problems and to solve them by himself without being influenced by this or that vested interest? While there is so much of 'progress' made in computer technology, man seems to have neglected the science that deals with advancement of mental capabilities.

The primary requisite

My object is not to condemn science and technology or modern research in various fields, but my plea is, let all these be utilised to serve the interests of peace, prosperity and happiness for mankind without exploitation of the one by the other. Let man-making education be made ideal by those in-charge of education and social welfare. When man-making education were to hold the field then the defects and disabilities seen in modern society would disappear in thin air.

Now without the basic requirement of health of body and mind, no progress is possible in any field. Is this the right kind of attention to the problem of the health of the body and the mind? On this question, the ancients in different parts of the world thought alike. People living in the modern world in different parts of the globe think in different ways: not only do they think differently, they even go to the extent of saying that 'outdated ideas' are not applicable today, thus casting away may time-honoured and time-tested truths as 'outdated', incompatible with modern thinking!

Another danger in the modern world is that the thought pattern of the majority alone is correct and what is put forward seriously by the minority is unscientific. And, the vested interests see to it that through mass propaganda, through newspaper, through television, Internet, etc., a majority is created in support of their stand.

A mind that unquestioningly accepts the views of others is a dull mind incapable of developing any further. Such a mind will accept the views of different vested interests and get confused on having different solutions, different suggestions on the same problem. What is known as mental conflict crops up in such a mind and whatever clarity might have been there earlier gets more and more clouded.

A mind, which has clarity in it, will neither accept nor reject others' views straightaway. A clear mind is ready to face each and every problem boldly and challengingly without any fear. It may take into account the data accumulated on the problem, but it would use its powers of discrimination, analysis and independent judgement to decide what is best. It will not even be swayed by what is known as the culture indigenous to the society to which the person belongs. A clear mind takes into account all data available both from the ancient sources as also from the modern to reach a final judgement.

Clarity of mind the *yogic* way

The ancients in the orient had gone deep into the subject and the science of yoga is the outcome of such deep research. By and large there are four systems of yoga advocated for liberating the mind from self-centredness or selfishness, prejudice, sin and sinful living. Clarity of thought is the basic feature common to all these four systems of yoga — *jnanayoga, rajayoga, karmayoga* and *bhaktiyoga*.

The disciplined way of life that one has to chart out for himself for treading the path of yoga — let it be any of the four systems referred above — is what endows the mind with clarity of thought. However laudable the disciplines advocated in these four types of yoga may be, to the science-oriented modern man, all such disciplines turn into an anathema and later he openly says: "We modern men are interested in earthly possessions, not in otherworldly pursuits."

Hence I will suggest some methodology, the adoption of which will enable the health-seeker to have clarity of thought and by stages develop clarity to the highest extent possible. The methodology suggested here is rational and suits one with a scientific temper of mind and this methodology does not involve the practice of any rigorous discipline of the *yogic* type.

All the three steps suggested here will help the health-seeker to achieve this object.

An abiding faith in the laws of life

Life is not created by man; it is endowed in him. Life is the gift of Mother Nature to every being, including man. So long as life is there in the body, the body will function as an organised whole with a set purpose directed by the eternal, immutable and inviolable laws of Nature.

As man cannot be there without life, he has to understand these laws to govern the proper working of his body and mind.

If man were to be something like a machine 'which is totally lifeless', wherein some screws, bolts, nuts, piston, etc. can be removed and replaced mechanically at will, it would have been a different picture. The mechanical laws, the laws of physics, the laws of chemistry can never apply *ipso facto* to the living being. Life is at a far higher plane, even something un-understandable; even the rationalist, the atheist cannot deny the existance of life.

Common sense decrees, therefore, that every human being must, if he wants to live healthy and devoid of chronic diseases or to recover radically from a diseased condition back to normalcy, than, accept to live in tune with the laws of life.

The laws of life and the principles and procedures flowing out of these laws have been fully elaborated in the science of natural hygiene (popularly known as Nature cure). There are ever so many therapies prevalent in the modern world. But none deals with this particular aspect which is the very basis of health.

Now understanding of the laws, principles and procedures referred to above has to be accompanied by rightful living in tune with the laws, etc. When one starts living this way his understanding becomes deeper, more thorough and more perfect. Such onward development of the understanding of the laws of Nature would by itself bring about clarity of mind.

To the one uninitiated in this science of health, the adoption of Nature cure involves the acceptance of the need to follow a disciplined way of life. The very word 'discipline' seems to be an anathema to many. However, I plead with them with all humility: "Can there be progress, can there be development without the adoption of some kind of discipline?" Discipline that is advocated here is not a discipline imposed from outside. It is a discipline voluntarily undertaken by a person with full understanding of its implications for improving one's health progressively.

When one adopts Nature cure as a way of life with a clear objective towards the goal of better and better health (both at the physical and mental levels), the requisite base for clarity of mind gets already built in the person. Such a person is not swayed by any propaganda that is carried on by others.

Perfecting the 'mode of surrender' to Mother Nature

Where physics melts into the thin air of metaphysics, a scientist stops and wonders as to what lies beyond his research. As one starts living in tune with the laws of life understandingly, there comes a stage of wonderment. The law of cause and effect, which in the physical world can more or less be easily understood by all, is applied here in a subtle way. The order found in the organisation of the human body, the spirit of symbiosis among its various organs, the purposeful direction in the human body, when analysed deeply, to understand the nature of law-giver, leads us to the Ordainer. The person concerned surrenders himself totally to the Ordainer as he knows that under the law of cause and effect, he can do actions but the effect, i.e. the result, comes from the Ordainer. Surrender is not prostration to anyone; it is reaching a point of satisfaction;

33

it is maturity. By following Nature cure man seeks physical and mental health as a blessing from Mother Nature. He seeks the grace of Mother Nature, thereby totally surrendering himself and be able to visualise her form fully, and enjoy that bliss.

To such a staunch follower of natural hygiene, Mother Nature says: "The duty cast on thee is to follow the law. Through such following thou hast taken refuge in me. Thou hast surrendered thyself to me. Now it is the duty cast on me to perfect the clarity in thee." And, she does it.

Freedom from fear

When the mind is obsessed with fear, it is likely to be confused. It would have no courage whatever to face the situation that is causing the fear. There can be no clarity of mind in such a situation.

Clarity of the mind is needed all the time. However, when there is a problem, which creates fear in others, the mature mind does not get unnerved by the 'apparent immensity' of the problem. The graver the situation the more attention is required to deal with it. It may not be practicable to develop absolute fearlessness that is talked about in the higher realms of philosophy. But fearlessness can be developed by the individual in facing some fear-causing situations. The immature mind is full of doubts and fears on practically every issue. The person having such an immature mind will continuously weaken his nervous and glandular systems through subjection to these fears.

Maturity of mind, that capability of the mind to go through life with calm composure, that capability of the mind where the person can squarely face even a thorny problem or issue, has to be developed if a higher level of health is the objective of the person.

The solution to the problem lies within the problem, deep inside the problem and not outside it. Go on analysing the problem realistically and continue your efforts to reach the root of the problem. The moment the solution is sighted, the problem ceases to exist. That ability to analyse the problem deeply to its root is proof enough that the individual concerned is sincere in facing his problem. To seek solutions from others, to meekly accept their solutions is not a safe method to adopt. When one starts acting upon the solution suggested by others, doubts and fears creep in on whether the solution would really solve the problem.

Hence, the safe method is to apply the yardstick of truth to judge whether or not the answer/solution is correct. Patients suffering from chronic and advanced chronic diseases submit themselves meekly to the treatment that is foisted on them. But theirs is only passive participation. Where one is only passively applying his mind, he will be restless, tormented by doubts and fears. For the health-seeker I recommend adoption of the principle of dynamic direction, that is, whatever health-promoting/restorative methods he adopts should all be 'directed from within'. That direction must be dynamic and fearless.

Such dynamic direction becomes possible only when the person is fully convinced of the soundness of the philosophy behind the methods he adopts. In other words, these should be knowledge-oriented methods. To be able to undertake the only sane and safe health-restoration methods which are in tune with the laws of life, one must have a thorough understanding of the principles of unity of disease, unity of health and disease, unity of food and medicine, unity of cause and unity of treatment and above all, the working of the law of cause and effect. Such a thorough understanding on the part of the health-seeker makes him follow the principle of vital economy and the principle of non-violence. He follows this path fearlessly for he knows that the law of cause and effect could never be wrong.

The self-discipline involved in following this path to health would progressively strengthen his mind and add to the 'iron to the will' and through this method, clarity of mind can be developed.

The sincere Nature cure follower knows that the only way to add grit to the mind is by 'feeding' his mind through practice of virtues like simplicity, equanimity, generosity, integrity, adaptability and the like. As his mind is nurtured through the regular observance of such virtues in daily life, he finds himself in a situation where the 'common ideas and influences' do not affect him in any manner.

Some persons may feel that the modern worldly conditions do not allow a person to develop the level of clarity of mind that has been set about as the ideal. Such persons, if they happen to be unhealthy, can follow the principles of Nature cure and benefit to the extent they deserve. Let them not resort to any system that only gives symptomatic relief; what is needed is a radical cure by observing vital economy.

Mind Management

The mind is not a bodily organ like the lungs, the heart, the kidneys or even the brain.

The brain is mistaken by some to be the mind, whereas it is not really so. The brain is a part of the central nervous system from where the nerves originate and reach all over the body. The mind is just a tool or instrument through which the organs in the body can be made to help the intellect, the *viveka* or power of discrimination to choose the right method and work thereupon.

What the mind is, where it is located inside the body, how perversions of the mind take place, how the mind can be controlled on proper lines, etc. are questions, which are far beyond the ken of science. But for that reason one cannot say that one need not concern oneself with the topic under discussion. The mind is the power mechanism through which all activities are directed and carried out through the medium of the physical organism in different ways.

A body without the mind behind it is an idiot, incapable of sensible functioning. It is not possible to imagine a mind without the body. The two together make a human being. And behind the two is the propelling spirit — call it the soul, the *jeeva*, the *atman*, anything you like. The body, as it is, is inert. The mind too is inert really speaking. It is the propelling spirit behind it that gives power to both.

If anyone wants to know, then learn in depth the relevant facts about the mind, its mysteries and its control, the scriptures can help him. In the scriptures of the orient, the *rajayoga* of Maharishi Patanjili reveals these factors threadbare.

There is a subtle body behind the gross body. Whereas the gross body is visible to everyone, the subtle body, known as *sukshma shareera* has in it, so says the *Yoga Shastra*, the *antahkarana*, the inner workshop. The mind is a part of *antahkarana*, the whole thing being totally invisible — all having the emanating power from within. The mind enables the human being to delve into the pros and cons of every issue/problem/question before him/her. Let it be noted that the function of the mind is only this. It is not the deciding factor. The mind has in it some defects/disability factors. If in any person such disabilities or disturbing factors are predominant, the power of the mind to delve into the pros and cons will not be present as the body has too much of foreign matter in it to work ideally. A mind with such defects/weaknesses is more of a liability than an asset for the person.

There is in the *antahkarana*, the *buddhi* (perhaps the nearest synonym in English is 'intellect'), which is the deciding factor. The *buddhi* is the judge. The *buddhi* decides after taking some useful tips from *viveka* or the power of discrimination. *Vichara,* the power of enquiry, enables the person to look at the distant goal and not miss it.

When dealing with the worldly matters while managing the worldly affairs, the *buddhi* — which is the heart of the *antahkarana* — has to be brought into full play. *Buddhi* must have correct background data from *viveka, vichara,* etc.

Unfortunately for the modern man, all this knowledge is more of a closed book. Just like guided democracy, the person straight from childhood is being 'guided' through the so-called educational system and the functioning of his intelligence is more at the superficial level, not taking into account the eternal values that are guiding life from within.

For ideal health, a health-seeker should go deeper into the subject. And that is what is being attempted in this chapter. The steps given here are based on hygiene, the science of health, which can be understood by any person and practised in daily life with adoption of some discipline in living. What is stated here is actually 'buddhi management'.

What does control of mind mean?

The word 'control' does not mean suppression. The mind, if it is not subjected to any code of sensible discipline, is immature. An immature mind would not allow the *buddhi* to function properly. The immature mind reacts, but reacts without devoting full thought to the problem/issue/question on hand. An immature mind is restless and a restless mind is wasting its innate power. It vainly hopes for the unattainable, for, to attain the desired goal one must put in honest and sincere effort, which the person with an immature mind is incapable of. The term control of mind simply means directing the powers behind the mind sensibly so that the weaknesses that predominate at the immature stage are cleared away. The controlled mind is mature enough, and the mature mind would allow the *buddhi* to function, guided by *viveka* and *vichara*. *Buddhi*, which is in fact the charioteer who guides the chariot (man's body) through his lifetime, ensures that the horses (sense organs) apparently take the chariot on the right road. It is *buddhi* management with the power of discrimination and enquiry playing a dominant role in guiding *buddhi*.

Two dominant forces

Let it be noted that behind every person there are two dominant forces (not equally strong in all) guiding the life of man. One is the superior mind and the other is the inferior mind. The former exercises its sober, restraining influence to see that the person does not succumb to evil influences. The latter permits the person to lead a life as he pleases and as the people around live.

Where a person is literally controlled by his inferior mind, the powers of discrimination, enquiry, analysis, etc. are not at all allowed to function. Life is lived in a routine way. It is this section of humanity that lays itself open to various diseases/disabilities affecting the body and the mind. As the superior mind is never allowed to function, subjects like Nature cure do not appeal to them as worth studying or worth following.

On the other hand, where the superior mind exercises its role (through *buddhi* management) the inferior mind is made to realise its limitations fully and start behaving sensibly on future occasions.

What is ultimately good for man may look unpleasant at the beginning and difficult to follow. What is ultimately bad for man may look quite rosy in the beginning and easy to follow. Where *buddhi* management is in force, the person concerned is not fooled by the apparent difficulties; if the *buddhi* indicates that a particular path is right, the person firmly follows it, whatever be the apparent difficulties.

The restraining forces appear to be harsh on modern man seeking to limit his pleasure-seeking instincts. These restraining forces seek to isolate man from the majority. The one with the immature mind feels 'insecure' when he is 'pushed' into the minority.

The dance-drama depicted by the devils appears to be alluring indeed. The allurements, the temptations offered by these devils aping the angles, so, present the law of cause and effect in a very perverted manner that the effectiveness of the law of dual effects is totally denied by the actors of this dance-drama. As the suggestions put forward to the audience by the actors in this drama appear to be easy to adopt, requiring no self-restraint and as these promise enjoyment of worldly pleasures, the ones with the immature mind fall easy prey to the devils masquerading as man's beneficiaries.

While the above seems to hold a vast majority of modern mankind in its grip, the rest who care for the fundamentals and keep the law of dual effects always before their minds shun the philosophy, the theory, that wrong living can be made safe through modern scientific appliances.

What has been presented above depicts the two dominant forces by the side of every man and how the discerning individual can swim through this dangerous river with sharks and crocodiles on every side, on to safety on the ship of hygiene.

Mind management is the art of keeping the mind unaffected by the allurements, the temptations, by the evil forces. The restraining force, which essentially comes from the *buddhi* backed by *viveka* and *vichara*, is to the sensible man the redeemer, but for which he would have been drowned in the ocean of disease, distress, and dismay.

Natural hygiene, the redeemer

The science of natural hygiene containing the cumulative wisdom of many thinking men and women from all times and climes shows the ideal way to health to those unfortunate ones who are already in the grip of some disease or the other.

The moment one shows his willingness to understand the fundamentals of natural hygiene, half the problem of mind management is overcome. Gain this half this way and take steps to gain the other half by following the suggestions below for effective mind management:

Like your work

Everyone in the world has to do some work regularly every day which happens to be the same, day after day. The one who wants to progress in the art of mind management should start liking his daily work. Let him like his work almost to the point of considering his work as worship of God. Let him plan his work. Let him do it methodically, systematically in a spirit of dedication. Let not his daily work make him feel bored. Let not daily work be done in a tense way. Let him remember that the sense of fulfillment arising out of work well done is a great factor in building up his physical and mental health.

Learn to relax

While work is a basic need of living, let not the one who wants to be perfect in the art of mind management know that workaholism is as bad as, if not worse than, alcoholism. Let every day be divided in different sectors — one for work, one for relaxation, one for perfecting oneself internally, etc.

When one relaxes one can take to constructive hobbies. The term relaxation need not be taken as synonymous with idling one's time. Getting away from one's regular professional work to learn music, practise art or sculpture or painting or lose oneself in poetry, if one has the aptitude for it is relaxation. When one relaxes this way for two or three hours, he will enjoy the benefits of real relaxation. It is this spell of relaxation taken every day that will add grit to his *buddhi*.

Keep away from the multitude

Let the discerning person realise that greatness lies in choosing an ideal and working towards it. Let the 'ideal' be a noble one, which could keep the mind happy all the time. Ideals grow up only in solitude. Hence, let the one seeking to perfect the art of *buddhi* management keep himself in solitude for a little time every day. In fact, the ideal for adoption is to feel the blessings of solitude even when one happens to be in a multitude.

Develop serenity

As during the life-time of everyone there are bound to be spells of agony, distress and the like, the one who has learnt the art of mind management should, with the aid of philosophical formulae learnt by him earlier from different sources, keep himself detached from the surrounding turmoil, which is affecting everyone else around.

Mind management—a prerequisite to health

This book is meant to help the health-seeker in keeping the internal body ecology in as ideal a state as practicable. Very often one is faced with questions as to what one can do in the face of so many unhygienic factors around him. If one cannot get away from such an atmosphere, if one is imprisoned therein, the way to detachment described in this book can keep him in fairly good health, physically and mentally.

However difficult the path indicated here might appear, there is no alternative to it. Let the total approach be adopted all the time.

Sensible Control over Sense Organs

The sense organs

The human being has ten sense organs designed for knowing what is going on around him and for enabling him to move about, and perform various actions. In Sanskrit language these ten sense organs are termed as *indriyas*. Of the ten sense organs, five are known as sense organs of perception or *jnanendriyas*. These are the skin or the sense organ of touch which enables the human being to know the state of the weather around, as also to feel the sense of pressure (if any) exerted upon him from outside; the eyes, which are the organs of vision, informing the human being of what is going on around him; the ears, which enable the human being to hear what is communicated to him by others as also for getting awareness of anything likely to cause harm or injure his person; the tongue or sense of taste, which enables the human being to differentiate between what is good or bad for him so that he may have his daily diet on sensible lines; the nose, which is the sense organ of smell enabling man to know which smell is pleasant, which is irritating and which is obnoxious or nauseating.

The other five sense organs of action or *karmendriyas* are:

- the tongue — the organ of speech enabling the human being to vocalise and communicate his thoughts and ideas to others around;

- the hands — these are meant to enable the human being to take in his food and drinks, to put his thoughts on paper, and various acts which are essential for carrying out the pursuits of life as also those of livelihood;
- the feet — these enable the human being to move about here and there to meet the various requirements;
- the anus — this is the sense organ performing the very useful function of letting out the faecal matter from within the bowels; and
- the reproductive organ — this organ which starts becoming active on reaching the adult stage and continues to be so during the fertile period, enabling the male/female to have healthy progeny.

If the above sense organs were not there in the human body, there could have been no human being as such. Each one would be lying in a corner like a cabbage, the carrot or some other vegetable or fruit. These sense organs enable the human being to act as living beings, living purposefully and leading an ideal-oriented life.

The inner director

The organs form part of the gross body or *sthoola shareera*. But what makes them do their work is directed from within, in what is known as the subtle body or *sukshma shareera* of man. This 'inner mechanism' is actually the *indriya–* technically known as *antahkarana* in the scriptures — the inner director. The vital reserve or *prana shakti* enables the human being to live through his span of life in the *antahkarana*. The individual soul, *jeevatma*, is the power which enables the *antahkaran* to do its directional work.

The spiritual outlook of man and his understanding of the concept of life are in fact the twin forces which steer man through life. In a special sense, it is this aspect of human personality which enables him to take the desired and desirable work through the various *indriyas* and helps him to desist from engaging the *indriyas* in undesirable channels, which bring out the beast in man and make him subhuman.

This brief interpolation at this stage is meant to stress the fact that the secrets of 'man, the unknown' are to be probed into thoughtfully, seriously and dedicatingly if man were to experience true happiness while living in this world and enable him to realise the aim and purpose of human life.

Let us revert to the earth level and learn

- how to steer through one's life with all the sense organs in good health all the time. And conversely,
- how an individual with dull understanding, imitates some people around, not having any sensible idea of how to direct this chariot through one's life.

The main purpose here is not to educate oneself spiritually but to so manage one's sense organs as to help them and in return be helped by them to be able to live a near ideal level of health.

Observance of the principle of vital economy

If in any individual the *indriyas* 'happen to be' rebellious, if consequently the person goes on indulging in so-called sense pleasures — maybe of taste or smell or sound or sex, etc. — the vital power would be tremendously wasted. The consequence would be that the concerned person would feel vital depletion in all the organs.

The writer feels that this state of serious vital depletion is what is called Acquired Immunity Deficiency Syndrome (AIDS) of the modern days.

What could enable a sensible person to keep himself safe without falling in an abyss of vital depletion, what could enable him to desist from rushing down the slippery path, are his mind and the intellect or the *buddhi*. The mind and the intellect are not physical organs in the human body. These again are in the subtle body.

Unless and until man takes some sensible steps to channelise his mental energies towards a constructive purpose, unless and until he sharpens his *buddhi*, the future will be bleak indeed. Mere worldly status or monetary advantage can render no help whatever to such a person. Let it be realised that the human being is not a mere body but that there is a triple unity of body, mind and spirit behind him. Man's welfare rests solely on one vital point, and that is, he should care for his body without injuring the structural integrity of his organs, without impairing the functional efficiency of different systems in the human body; caring for his mind by taking vigilant, sensible steps to clear the dross therefrom so that the mind can furnish the proper data to the intellect, the *buddhi*, to enable the latter to take the right decision on every question and; to spiritually care for the ultimate welfare of the *jeevatma* within by observing the spiritual concepts enshrined in the scriptures.

What has been explained in the preceding paragraphs represents the total approach towards the ideal or the near ideal health. Where special care is not endowed on the points mentioned above and to the extent the care will be lacking, the *indriyas* will rebel. The more uncontrollable the rebellion the more the mischief. The lesser the rebellion the lesser the mischief.

Every person in the world wants to be healthy. Maybe the spiritual *sadhana* referred to earlier may look to the common man to be impossible of adoption and he may question whether there are other sensible ways to keep himself (along with his *indriyas*) healthy all through life. What follows is meant for the common man.

Here is the solution offered to the common man not acquainted with the intricacies of the oriental philosophy. Here is the three-fold programme for the common man.

Unshakable or firm faith in natural hygiene

The common man wants to be healthy all through his life. If he is really earnest about his desire, he must know the laws and principles governing human health, physical and mental. The *materia medica* may not at all be able to help him in this direction for this is mostly a list of inedible poisons. He ought to know that there is a *materia hygienica*, a product of Mother Nature that has fashioned his body and given him the needed life power, enabling him to live in this world sensibly.

The common man must make effort to understand the rules of hygiene, which are based upon the laws referred to earlier. He must understand them in depth. These rules of hygiene are fully codified and elaborated in the science of natural hygiene or basic Nature cure.

Having understood their practical importance, the person should start living hygienically. If he is occasionally forced to violate the rules of hygiene, he should at the earliest stage repent for his mistake and set himself on the right path. Sincerity is the key word, which would enable him to progress rightly.

However 'popular and fashionable' the so-called social habits in society be, man must apply the yardstick of hygiene in every case and refrain from indulgence in such habits. Imitation is weakness and nothing else.

Understanding natural hygiene and following the rules prescribed therein for the sole purpose of keeping oneself healthy will specially tone up his nervous and glandular systems to enable him to control his mind in the right direction. The discipline

49

involved on this chosen path would tantamount to *buddhi* yoga and by taking to this *buddhi* yoga he will reject all remedies; he will be totally free from the twin evils of escapism and opportunism.

Living this way of life would mean that he has surrendered himself to Mother Nature who is *shakti* or power incarnate to God, the *shaktiman,* and the origin of that power.

Surrender to the ultimate reality

The common man going through the travails of worldly life is capable of this surrender and will not fail in discharging his worldly duties and responsibilities. Let it be understood clearly that one can go through worldly life and yet progress spiritually, step by step.

The term 'surrender to God' implies that the person concerned weans himself away from the idea of 'doer-ship', feels that he is only an agency through which actions are being done. He is also free from the idea of 'enjoyer-ship.' No doubt he will get the right reward for his action. But he will not be worried that the reward is much less than what he expected to have. He is always satisfied with the results obtained through his actions, there being no dissatisfaction in him.

Adoption of this attitude of mind will keep his mind calm and unruffled.

Total freedom from fear

When one imagines that insecurity is staring him in his face he is gripped by fear. And when he is so subjected to fear, he becomes unable to face the problem/issue on hand. To feel helpless in such a situation can only add to the misery of man.

Is there a sensible plan which could be adopted by the common man to free himself from fear totally so that he can face any situation with confidence and work out the solution in a proper manner?

The solution of problem/issue is within the problem itself. The deeper one goes into the problem, the more he thrashes the issue involved, the clearer will be the picture before him. Such a deep analysis will lead to a state where the problem will cease to exist and that will be its solution. Let us apply this precept in every case. And when, as a result of understanding arrived through such analysis is clear before our mind, there ought to be no fear in facing that issue/problem. The more we work on these lines on every issue/problem on hand, the more mature the mind will become.

Let us apply this modus operandi in relation to the problem of disease. Instead of meekly accepting the general view that germs/viruses/microbes are behind the causation of a disease or that every disease has to be fought through specific drugs prescribed by a qualified physician, let the common man analyse what disease is, why he is suffering from it and how he can get a radical cure. Let him realise that he is not the first person to get disease in the world. That many, many people before him have had illnesses and that quite many of them have radically cured themselves by adopting methods not generally accepted as right ones.

The mental persistence of man in finding out 'precedents' where people had cured themselves radically will strengthen his mind. As he gets busy in finding out the 'precedents', he will come across the science of natural hygiene; the science of health based upon the eternal, immutable and inviolable laws of life.

Such a persistent effort in understanding the very basis of the problem before him will endow fearlessness in him. This is known as *sagyana nirbhayata*, fearlessness arising out of a clear understanding of the problem at hand. Let the same method be applied to every problem/issue, maybe something unrelated to health or maybe related to problems concerning one's livelihood.

After all the problems/issues which one has to face could be listed out and one may seek to get fully informed of all the relevant facts about such problems/issues. The reader is asked to develop *sa-gyana nirbhayata* in relation to such problems/issues that may arise in future too.

In one's life there may arise unforeseen situations. The question is whether one could have fearlessness in facing such problems too.

There is the power of discrimination, *viveka*, dormant in the *antahkarana* of man. This power will be dormant so long as it is not utilised in the proper manner in one's daily life. I suggest that every person should utilise this power of discrimination in dealing with even common day-to-day problems/issues. Let every action of man be done after devoting a little serious thought to it, after applying one's power of discrimination. Let no action – however minor or routine it may look – be done impulsively without devoting such thought. Observance of this direction will sharpen the power of discrimination in man and with the help of such sharpened discrimination, one can face even unexpected situations that may arise in one's life here or there. This is what the writer would call *viveki nirbhayata*, that is, developing the state of fearlessness by sharpening one's power of discrimination.

There is one still another state of fearlessness, other than the one described above, and that is a state where one gets absolutely fearless. This state of fearlessness, which could be termed as *ishwarnishtha nirbhayata*, is fearlessness arising out of one's identification with that Supreme Power, that is behind the entire universe. Where there is total devotion in a person, he gets into a state of mind when he feels all his personal interests are being suitably looked after by the Higher Being, that he has nothing to fear in this world. History is replete with ideal personages who had reached this stage of *ishwaranishtha nirbhayata*.

Having outlined rather briefly the three types of fearlessness for the benefit of the reader, the writer will plead that at least the lowest type of fearlessness, the *sa-gyana nirbhayata,* may practically be put into use by every man. Even in this state of fearlessness the mind is clear, mature and free from base desires that trouble the immature minds of the people.

Let earnest effort be made to practise the first stage of fearlessness. Then only can one prepare himself for the other two stages. Sincere effort with total humility in one's mind would pay enormous dividends. Reference is made here to the need for humility in the person as the one who does not have this quality and who consequently feels 'proud' of his earlier achievement(s) cannot make any progress in the matter. His very egoism would hinder his progress.

Let the common man practise natural hygiene in his daily life. Let him clearly realise that there is a Supreme Power behind this grand show that is known as the world and that it is that power that directs the events in his daily life too. Let him develop at least the first stage of fearlessness referred to above. Let this programme be effectively put through with all sincerity. If this effort is made, the common man can control his mind. And, with that controlled mind with its great potential power behind, it can enable him to live better.

Success cannot be achieved in a day. Let sincere practice be adopted in following the above mode of action. In course of time the maturity of mind will be reached; the state of fearlessness can be developed. The progress will be step by step and let persistence and patience be the key words in the pursuit of this ideal.

Practical tips to keep sense organs in good shape

Here are some practical tips to act as 'effective brakes' and to be applied in directing the sense organs on proper lines.

The skin

- **Desirable:** Train the skin sensibly to bear the changes in weather. Do not indulge in overdressing on the plea that the weather is very cold. While exposure to too much of heat/too much of cold is definitely against the interests of one's health, one should, while adopting a hygienic diet and taking an air-bath daily, train his skin in putting up with the vagaries of weather.

  Undesirable: Indulgence in overdressing, seeking to live in air-conditioned apartments all the time and carelessness in matters concerning one's diet and development of fear that the cold air outside would cause the common cold, pneumonia, etc.

- **Desirable:** Realisation of the truth that clothing is just for comfort and not for fashion, that is current in the society outside.

  Undesirable: Developing fascination for the latest in fashion in matters of dress.

- **Desirable:** Having sunbath in mild sunlight for some time every day as and when practicable, as sunlight furnishes the needed nutrition to the skin.

  Undesirable: Abstinence from even a little exposure in mild sunlight, using dark, deep coloured clothes and wearing them tightly over the skin.

- **Desirable:** Keeping away from the use of chemicals, beauty aids, artificial scents and the like, as everyone of these irritates the skin and adversely affects its normal functions as a sense organ.

  Undesirable: Indulgence in beauty aids on the plea that that is the latest in fashion.

- **Desirable:** Let the sensation of touch over the skin be kept to the minimum (the intention is to keep the sense organ of skin at the maximum possible health level).

Undesirable: Developing a craving and uncontrollable desire for experiencing the sensation of what an individual considers to be 'pleasure for the skin' and repeated indulgence in such pleasures beyond permissible limits of hygiene, moral and social precepts prescribed for them.

The eyes

- Desirable: Let the eyes be engaged in reading/writing or other work without producing visual fatigue.

  Undesirable: Engaging the eyes on work under a dim light or under very bright light; engaging oneself in television viewing to the extent of becoming an addict to the habit (as radiation would seriously impair health); looking at things with evil intentions in mind, with greed, avarice and the like; engaging oneself in working on mechanical instruments for a long time daily involving fixing of tiny screws and other fittings to such instruments.

- Desirable: Adoption of right posture in sitting/standing while one is engaged in reading, writing, etc.

  Undesirable: Adoption of wrong posture in sitting or standing while at work (as this will tend to cause curvatures in spine and sometimes even in the bones of hip or the leg).

- Desirable: Where practicable (even occasionally) standing sometime and looking at a natural scenery and losing oneself in it.

  Undesirable: Mistaking them to be entertainment or relaxation, spending time watching rock 'n roll dance or scenes likely to stimulate one's sex urge.

- **Desirable:** Engaging oneself (within reasonable limits) in hobbies like painting, drawing, sculpture, etc. Adopting the right posture in sitting/standing while one is on such work.

  Undesirable: Engaging oneself in so-called hobbies, which are likely to stimulate or irritate the different sense organs, or in so-called (unproductive) hobbies wasting one's time and energy.

- **Desirable:** So planning one's daily routine that engages the eyes on work/hobbies under pleasant natural light.

  Undesirable: Work till very late at night under electric light.

- **Desirable:** Devoting hygienic care in preserving eyesight all through life.

  Undesirable: Start wearing spectacles even from an early age and use of contact lenses, rubbing the eyes and often use of collyrium, antimony ground into fine powder or any similar stuff in the eyes.

The ears

- **Desirable:** The ears are meant to be engaged on listening to sweet sound, sweet speech, etc.

  Undesirable: Exposing one's ears to harsh speech or to terrific noise or even to persistent noise created by the working of machines (known as noise pollution); lending one's ears to someone who uses foul language, indulging in abuse or scandalising.

- **Desirable:** Devoting hygienic care to the maintenance of health of the outer ear, including the eardrum and concerned nerves.

  Undesirable: Under the wrong impression that one is 'caring for the ears' means putting oil of some kind inside the ears and trying to cleanse the ears in the wrong way (which may even lead to the damage of the ear-drum).

Sensation of taste (the tongue)

- **Desirable:** Hygienically selecting one's food to be taken in moderation, and satisfying the sense of taste to the desired extent.

  Undesirable: Influenced mainly by the social atmosphere around by taking in of products having no health-value whatever and 'enjoying' the 'taste' occasioned thereby.

- **Desirable:** Consumption of natural foods only when hungry and that too moderately, chewing every morsel.

  Undesirable: Lunching and munching all through the day.

- **Desirable:** Taking in of food not more than twice a day and ensuring that food is taken in only when some physical rest could be had after eating.

  Undesirable: Taking three or more meals/or fast foods under the wrong impression that the food is the source of energy.

- **Desirable:** Taking in of natural foods of a mild *satvik* taste.

  Undesirable: Indulging in highly condimented, spiced, fried foods; indulging in use of processed foods manufactured, tinned, bottled, canned stuff; developing a liking for meat, chicken, fish, etc. under the impression that one is 'strengthening' his nerves by going in for synthetic vitamins, synthetic minerals, so-called tonics, etc.

- **Desirable:** As and when absolutely necessary, taking fresh juices of raw vegetables, seasonal fruits in moderate quantity.

  Undesirable: Addiction to tea, coffee, cola drinks, etc. as also to products like beer, whisky, etc. (forgetting the truth that water is the only real drink and that all the stuffs mentioned are poisons).

The nose

- **Desirable:** As Nature has designed the nose for helping man to keep away from smells of highly irritating or obnoxious nature, developing the needed discrimination for knowing what is hygienic and good for the person; learning to enjoy a sweet fragrance emanating from the flowers and herbs but taking care not to be ensnared by such fragrance.

  Undesirable: Irritating the nasal membrane by use of products like snuff, etc. or the nicotine fumes emitted by cigarettes or irritating the nasal membrane through indulgence in the *neti kriya* (*jala neti, sutra neti, ghrita neti*) recommended by some so-called experts; working in factories/other places where the stench of chemicals or chemical vapours is in the atmosphere around; exposing one's nostrils to air with unhygienic constituents mixed in it.

- **Desirable:** Taking hygienic care for the maintenance of physical health and ensuring that the nostrils do not get clogged by phlegm or any other foreign matter.

  Undesirable: Mistaking the development of common cold and other consequent catarrhal disorders as 'disease' to be fought off; resorting to drug treatment or the *yogic* treatment. (The nose is to be kept clean through natural living and not through the so-called cleansing).

- **Desirable:** To enable the nasal mucus membranes to be in their natural healthy state by regular daily practice of *pranayama* in a non-violent manner.

  Undesirable: Indulgence in the performance of *hatha yogic pranayama* like *bhastrika, seetali, seetakari, bhramari,* etc. as these are definitely far beyond the capacity of the average man and hence result in damaging the very structure of all parts of the respiratory system, including the nostrils.

The organ of speech (the tongue)

- **Desirable:** Taking proper care to convey one's ideas only after devoting thoughtful deliberation over what is to be communicated (except where the speech relates to purely routine matters).

  Undesirable: Indulging in violent outbursts, stimulated by one's impulse; talking incoherently with one's mind in deep anguish or agony.

- **Desirable:** Conveying one's ideas in a pleasant language even when one is not in agreement with the other person and even where a criticism of the other party is to be conveyed.

  Undesirable: Violent criticism couched in rude language.

- **Desirable:** Observing politeness in speech when talking to elders but conveying one's ideas or basic desire in unmistakable terms.

  Undesirable: Indulgence in impolite or undiplomatic language to convey one's strong disagreement with the other.

- **Desirable:** Factually presenting the truth or true situation where it is not likely to cause any harm to another's health, physical or mental.

  Undesirable: Indulgence in speech of a nature likely to seriously disturb others around.

- **Desirable:** Controlling oneself and even preferring to keep silent when talking is likely to upset the atmosphere around (but keeping one's face fairly serene and calm without the facial appearance conveying one's strong disagreement).

  Undesirable: Not caring for maintenance of proper inter-personal relationship, expressing oneself in rude language (under the impression that one is honestly conveying what is and what is not to be done).

- **Desirable:** Setting up right standards in one's speech and making everyone around know on the underlying sincerity and devotion to truth in the speaker.

  Undesirable: Fashioning one's speech which is impelled by undesirable qualities like escapism, opportunism, etc.
- **Desirable:** Thoughtfully choosing the words employed in one's communication to achieve the twin objectives of good inter-personal relationship and setting right the psychological disturbance prevalent in the atmosphere.

  Undesirable: Impulsive speech impelled by one's impulses without devoting any thought to the consequences that may follow.
- **Desirable:** Thoughtfully restraining oneself where occasions so demand and preferring to keep silent.

  Undesirable: Losing one's emotional poise and giving vent to such upsets in one's speech in an undesirable manner.
- **Desirable:** Ensuring that one's mode of speech does not in any way inhibit the inward flow of information or facts.

  Undesirable: Employment of a language that is likely to create antagonism or disturbed relationship, resulting in total breakage of the relationship.
- **Desirable:** As one's mode of speech is fashioned more by the culture in the individual, practising spiritual *sadhana* like attentively listening to the advice of elders and saints and by intensive study of scriptures containing noble truths; thoughtfully listening to the mode of speech of respected elders and fashioning one's own mode of speech in a similar manner.

  Undesirable: Rejecting the need to learn from elders/scriptures and shaping one's mode of speech more through watching/observation of television, movies, etc.

The hands

- **Desirable:** Employing the hands in doing productive work or in such work as would enable the person to improve his knowledge or learning.

  Undesirable: Using the hands for doing mechanical work but taking no interest in the work itself and with no job satisfaction.

- **Desirable:** Clapping the hands in a gentle manner to convey one's joy or pleasure at a given moment.

  Undesirable: Using the hand to beat another or to convey one's strong dislike of another; even insulting the other in the process.

- **Desirable:** As speaking and writing go together, employing the hand in writing what is desirable.

  Undesirable: Employing the hand in writing dirty language or drawing senseless figures 'enjoying some sensual pleasure in one's mind'.

- **Desirable:** Where one's professional interest so demands and where one wants to gain expertise in the profession using one's hands and the fingers thereof (as in *Bharatanatyam* dance and other classical dances) to express without actually speaking one's subtle thought, ideas and motives.

  Undesirable: Using the hands and fingers thereof purposelessly, even disturbing others around in the process.

- **Desirable:** Keeping the hands free from any tightness around it or around its fingers to ensure the maintenance of the tone of the nerves in the region.

  Undesirable: Using of tight gloves, even if made of cotton (gloves made of synthetic fibre being far more objectionable) to cover the hand.

- **Desirable:** When one's professional interest so demands, using one's fingers over the percussion producing musical instruments, etc. as non-violently as possible and just for the time needed and massaging the fingers of the hands thereafter to ensure proper relaxation of the nerves and blood flow.

   Undesirable: Using the fingers in operating the percussion producing musical instrument so violently that one's nerves get even injured in the process.

The feet

- **Desirable:** Keepings legs free from socks, sockets, cramping footwear, using only, where necessary, material made of cotton fibre and footwear made of leather and not of any synthetic material.

   Undesirable: Use of high heeled shoes or cramping footwear made of synthetic material like plastic, rubber, etc.; use of tight socks, sockets, etc.

- **Desirable:** Where one's professional interests so demand, use of legs in graceful movements as in classical dances as and when needed.

   Undesirable: Indulgence in rock 'n roll dance or similar dances of the violent type losing a lot of one's energy and taxing one's muscles in the process.

- **Desirable:** A daily walk (especially in the cool early morning hours), walking over grass where possible or over uneven ground so that the arch in the feet also gets the much-needed 'earth contact'.

   Undesirable: With no specific exercise given to the legs, standing over the same area for hours on end doing one's professional work (where such standing for long hours is imposed on a person, he should do corrective exercises like cycling in the air, both in the morning and evening).

- **Desirable:** Ensuring that the legs get enough and proper blood circulation by keeping them healthy and not allowing the deposition of unwanted fat over the thighs, etc.

    Undesirable: Living a sedentary life with no physical exercise whatever and living in a manner as to result in deposition of unwanted fat in the lower abdomen, the hip region, the thighs, etc.

- **Desirable:** Sitting with legs in a relaxed posture while one is at work.

    Undesirable: Sitting with one thigh pulled over the other or moving the legs or toes unnecessarily.

The anus

- **Desirable:** Proper maintenance of bowel health including that of the anus by living in tune with laws of life.

    Undesirable: Forcing the anal muscles to release the faecal matter from the bowels by application of mechanical pressure over the anus, the use of purgatives/laxatives, the use of the enema with plenty of water mixed with soap or glycerine, inserting one's fingers through the anus and removing the faecal matter therefrom.

- **Desirable:** Creating a bowel habit to evacuate the faecal matter once early in the morning and once by sunset time and sticking to the time as far as possible.

    Undesirable: Forcing the anus to retain the stools within, even after an urge is felt.

- **Desirable:** Keeping the anal region as cool as practicable.

    Undesirable: Sitting on padded chairs for long hours daily and wearing tight underclothing, causing heat and congestion in the region.

63

- **Desirable:** Keeping digestion alright so that no part of the digestive system (including the large intestine and the anus) is taxed. This is the 'assistance' that the anus seeks from man.

    Undesirable: Frequent expulsion of gas through the anus taxing the anal sphincters considerably.

The reproductive organs

- **Desirable:** As the abuse/misuse of this organ can even wreck one's constitution (which when once wrecked cannot be re-built), acquirement of the basic knowledge on sane and safe living through sensible control over the sex urge is to be prac-tised all through life.

    Undesirable: Mistaking that sex indulgence affords plea-sure to the individual, resort to such practices as masturbation in adolescence and early youth, attempt to 'enjoy' sex by read-ing sexy literature or engaging one's vision on sexy scenes or near nude dances, by developing a perverse attitude towards sex all the time, by dressing oneself in tiny dresses or any type of dress which can 'attract' other sex, by making ungraceful movements of the body with the sole purpose of enticing the other sex.

- **Desirable:** Following long-established conventions in regulat-ing one's conduct with the other sex, understanding the mean-ing and purpose behind such conventions.

    Undesirable: Refusing to recognise the wisdom of elders in society through whom such long-established social conventions have come into being; freely taking part in performances at night clubs, etc; indulging in the daily use of the so-called sex tonics and falsely imagining that one can live all through life in this manner.

- **Desirable:** Fully recognising the fact that healthy progeny is the reward of Mother Nature given to a person who does not waste his/her vitality through frequent indulgence in sex; leading one's married life happily by fulfilling all the duties imposed by social conventions on the husband/wife; limiting the sex contact as much as practicable (the husband can keep the wife satisfied, and *vice versa* too in ever so many other ways than through frequent indulgence in sex).

    Undesirable: Mistaking marriage as a free licence granted to one to indulge in sex as and when one likes; developing a craze for sex for most of the time.

- **Desirable:** Recognising that one's brain health goes hand in hand with the observation of *brahmcharya* in one's life, taking proper steps at every level to enable a person to progress more towards developing that state of mind wherein one can feel satisfied and happy through observance of *brahmacharya* to the greatest extent possible, even while one is living a married life.

    Undesirable: Casting the spiritual values away as outmoded, outdated; adoption of habits which can only make living literally miserable and trying to correct this internal misery through indulgence in stimulants, sedatives, drugs, etc., thus adding to this misery.

Effort to achieve the object of life

While each one has to go through the humdrum of worldly life, bearing the knocks and blocks therein, it is however meaningless to pull through the so-called problems and privations. Life must be lived with a purpose, with an objective in mind and there should be a constant endeavour towards the achievement of that objective. While at the physical level, man has to be healthy to keep himself happy and satisfied, at the super-mental level he should aim at achieving the peace that is beyond verbalisation. While many in the modern world may dismiss this objective as impossible of achievement, it is this very reason that the supposed impossibility of achievement or why the *dhira*, the valiant individual, should work towards it.

Of all the living beings on this planet the human being is the one gifted with various faculties and talents which are not to be found in lower species. Through sensible control over his sense organs the human being can reach higher and higher stages of mental quietude, the ultimate goal being perfection. What in Indian philosophy is known as *indriya nigraha* it means sensible control over sense organs listed above. Those who are not interested in the spiritual side of life — and there are very many in the modern world belonging to this category – can at least enjoy a very high level of mental health enabling them to make a solid contribution to the welfare of humanity as a whole. Let not the concept of *indriya nigraha* be dismissed as 'other worldly'. Greatness lies in working towards noble ideals, rising far, far above the pleasures of the flesh. Having the body of the human being with the mental equipment attached thereto, let man not only limit himself to the achievement of a disease-free life but aim at and work towards his ideal so that his very existence in this world will prove to be an asset for the entire humanity for all time to come. *Indriya nigraha* is the first step. The moment one achieves success in passing through this first step, his further passage will be clear to his mind. The inner man, the unknown man within the human body with tremendous faculties that are there within him will transform the very personality of the 'outer individual'. Let the ideal be kept in mind. Let the march onward to this ideal be helped by the friendly sense organs or *indriyas* which role these will assume when once they are sensibly controlled.

The one that fails to sensibly control one's sense organs is likely to be an abode of disease. The hints given here are intended to keep man healthy and there is no alternative method. Intake of drugs — the so-called medicines — cannot endow man with health.

A lot of vital energy is wasted through the sense organs indulging in worldly activities of one's liking. All this vital waste has to be prevented to make life healthy and happy.

Activity

In the days of yore when man's surroundings were natural, natural foods were available and everyone had to be somewhat active in the process of daily living as there were no machines and gadgets. In such circumstances the organs inside the human organism could not go haywire. The functions inside were fairly normal in practically all the cases.

In fact it is only when all the organs inside the organism are functioning systematically and doing their proper work can health be enjoyed.

The picture is quite different now. In modern days, with machines and gadgets galore, with refining of foods rampant everywhere and with no need to do anything physically, man's basic need of living is not being 'supplied'. And, this is one basic reason as to why the health level is falling in quite a large number of cases in the modern days. The problem is to be faced correctly. What is the solution?

Ensuring internal activity

A living body has to have proper internal activity — neither too much nor too little, and this balanced activity inside the organism is possible only when man is prepared to switch over to the adoption of a new lifestyle in tune with the principles of health. There is no other alternative available to man if he wants to be healthy.

A tense nervous system cannot be normalised through tranquillisers and the like. Already the nervous system is tense, i.e. unhealthy. Further use of tranquillisers can only make the nervous system more unhealthy.

Similarly a clogged bowel unable to eliminate the faecal matter daily is already weak and that is why it is not able to discharge its work. Use of purgatives and laxatives can only irritate the mucous membranes of the bowel and weaken it further.

Wrong living cannot be made safe by any drug therapy. In fact it is illogical to hold that certain remedies can make wrong living safe.

A sleepless individual is already suffering. To administer barbiturate (so-called sleeping pill) can only weaken his system, making sleep still more impossible. Common sense can clarify that drugs cannot normalise an abnormal or subnormal structure within. One can normalise an activity within only by changing his lifestyle.

Let the wise one so change his lifestyle, normalise the internal activities of the different organs and thus see that this much-needed basic need of living is made available to man. This is the solution that the science of natural hygiene puts before all health-seekers.

In modern times, however much one may live hygienically through diet reform, through sunbathing, through rhythmic breathing, etc., it may not be possible for the health-seeker to ensure that the skeletal muscles are kept active to the desired extent. This may happen to be a problem in many cases.

Mere restoration of normal functioning inside the organism may not be enough if there is no scope for activity of the skeletal muscles. Hence, to ensure normal activity for the skeletal muscles, man may have to do some exercise or take resort to some games like football, cricket, etc. If the skeletal muscles are not active, even the blood circulation would become sluggish affecting the health of the whole body. Hence, let some exercise be done regularly. Over-exercise is not recommended, lifting heavy weights is not advised, but enough exercise for all the skeletal muscles of the body is recommended.

Maintenance of normal functioning inside is a basic need of living. Where there is no scope in daily life for activity of the skeletal muscles, let exercise be done to ensure that the basic need is 'supplied' fully.

Every organ, every tissue in the body is to have its normal activity every day. Otherwise it would lose its efficiency and health. To ensure proper activity of every muscle in the body, exercise has to be done. To this extent exercise is not a tax on vitality.

If, however, anyone indulges in over-exercising ostensibly to build his musculature, if any one indulges too much in games that would definitely mean a tax on vitality, for the activity forced on musculature is not for supplying a basic need of living.

A few words on exercise

Exercise is of three types: (1) hygienic exercise, (2) educational exercise, and (3) corrective exercise.

The type of exercise referred to in the preceding paragraph is hygienic exercise, i.e. which would enable a person to maintain the hygienic condition within the organism. There cannot at all be any objection to this.

Educational exercise is resorted to by sportsmen with the main object of winning gold and silver medals in national or international sports events. To be able to achieve this rather extraordinary standard, they have to train themselves assiduously day after day. They apply their mind seriously to their programmes, trying to establish neuro-muscular co-ordination in their bodies. This type of exercise is needed by certain professionals taking part in sports events. This may well be a tax on vitality. But, if the concerned person wants to stick to his profession, he will have to take extraordinary care in observing the principle of vital economy very strictly in all other facets of life. Otherwise the health might suffer later.

Those who had adopted wrong posture while sitting, working, sleeping, etc. and as a consequence have developed spinal curvatures, etc. in their bodies could, before the curvature becomes unmanageable, take to corrective exercise to rectify the deformities.

Let it be noted that it is not only for correcting the curvature that corrective exercise is to be done, people who have to stand for long hours daily for doing their work may develop varicose veins in course of time. People who indulge in dance far beyond their physical capacity, straining themselves in performing the required movements of hands, legs, etc., may slowly and steadily develop flat feet. Corrective exercises have to be done for such cases to prevent the development of such deformities.

Those concerned should take to hygienic diet, improve their breathing, rectify their posture while sitting, etc. in addition to their specific corrective exercises. The principle of 'vital economy' cannot be ignored by anyone aiming to improve his health.

Quite apart from normalisation of internal functions, one has to ensure that his daily work in the outer world is done with care, attention and propriety. Such work may either be physical or mental. Whatever it may be, each one has to do his work.

Maybe such work may form a part of their regular official duty or their career. While such work is being done with a motive behind it, viz. to earn one's living and while that motive may be fulfilled through their earnings, let the health-seekers remind themselves that there is something beyond the monetary gains arising out of such work. If such work is done in the proper manner — as is explained here — such activity can improve one's health level slowly.

Let no one dislike his work. Where possible, change the type of work if you are dissatisfied with it. But this may not be practicable in all cases.

Have zest for your work. Even though you may be doing the same work every day in the same atmosphere, do not get bored. Look upon every day's work afresh and feel that you are contributing something to the nation's prosperity. Love your work, do your work as worship with all attention and devotion. If this attitude is adopted, especially the habit of looking at every day's work afresh, your efficiency will improve tremendously. Let the sense of fulfilment that you derive from the work that is well done make you happy. As efficiency will improve day by day, one will be able to work more in less time. Better set an example to shirkers who have no happiness in them and make them also take interest in their work fully.

Work: A basic need of living

Work done in the manner indicated above would steadily improve one's mental health and thus this basic need of living is a health-promoting factor. Work done by one in the outside world (apart from the functions inside one's organism and the exercise done by him daily) is also an activity. This activity is not only needed by the individual as his basic need of living but the work being done by lots of people in the society is what is keeping the society stable, rich, progressive. Let every worker feel that he is an asset to the nation and in order to do his work effectively day after day, let him carefully keep up his physical health as carefully as possible. Thus each one can ensure the nation's prosperity.

Completion of a piece of work is possible only when it is done methodically, systematically and orderly. Each piece of work is to be done this way in order to ensure that the worker does not create problems for others around him, especially where machines have to be handled in discharging one's daily work. Let the mechanism of the concerned machines be carefully kept in mind so that the machines do not go out of order.

Activity as a basic need of living is threefold — maintenance of internal functions inside the organism to the desired extent, performance of exercise to the extent needed and not more, and discharge of one's daily work efficiently, effectively and cheerfully.

Let this basic need be supplied by everyone and see what wonderful results arise out of the supply of this need.

Wisdom in Eating

In this scientific era of ours where every person is expected to adopt the scientific temper of mind and do actions after a thorough analysis of it, the pity is that most of mankind today is eating unwisely. In the books of nutrition adorning the shelves of all public libraries, sample data are there on nutritive elements in natural foods made available to man through the plant kingdom.

But the pity of pities is that no food is taken in, in its natural form today. Stale foods and junk foods are shoved in. Foods are refined, processed and tampered with. And, to add to the misery of man, the vitamins, minerals, salts, enzymes etc. are not available to man in their natural form. But these come to him through the shelves of chemist shops in a synthetic form. I am not for a moment admitting that what is told in the books dealing with the science of nutrition is fully correct.

The scientists aver that food is the source of energy behind the working of man's body. They have produced calorie tablets, which enjoin man that he should take in 'a specified quantum of food every day'. This aspect of science of nutrition is a travesty of facts and there is so much of disease the world over, simply because everyone happens to be calorie minded.

Around A.D. 1900 there was practically no science of nutrition as is known today. But the fact was that in those days all food was available to mankind in the form produced by Mother Nature.

There was far less disease in those days. Today the picture is totally different though we have accumulated a lot of knowledge through books on the science of nutrition.

Unless and until man happens to be wise in eating, he cannot maintain his health, he cannot improve his standard further. As for patients at present having certain disability in their body organisation, they cannot regain their health unless they happen to be wise in eating.

Everyone wants to feel energetic in life all the time. Hence, each one must know how this can be ensured all through life.

What makes the living organism work through its different systems, work as ideally as possible, what makes the different eliminatory organs in man carry on their activities faultlessly day after day, is the life power termed *prana shakti* in the Indian philosophy. Every health-seeker must clearly recognise what this *prana shakti* is, how not to spend it wrongly in his various actions, physical and mental, and how to ensure health and longevity through the observance of the principle of vital economy.

Let me at this stage list all the points on the essentials of nutrition, the observance of which constitute 'wisdom in eating'.

The three-fold classification of food

To enable him to know clearly which foods are health-promoting/health-restoring, each person should know the three-fold classification of food, viz. primary or positive foods, secondary or negative foods and denatured or devitalising foods. The third category is not actually deemed as natural foods but a mention of it has been made here as the market shelves are full of these and these are advertised through the mass media as 'energising foods'. The gullible ones are easily taken away by the alluring advertisements. Many of these happen to have within them synthetic flavours and synthetic colours. Many of them have chemical preservatives to enable them to have a long shelf-life. Many of them have additives in them. These are vital points which are kept away from public gaze.

Every natural food that has been tampered with (while processing, manufacturing or refining it) is unfit for human consumption as none of these can have any real health value whatever. These may stimulate man's taste buds and make him an addict to them, but no positive health value can be derived from any of these.

All manufactured foods, all processed foods, all synthetic food products, all tinned or bottled and packed foods, all fast foods, all refined foods come under the third category and the health-seeker is advised to keep away from these in his own interest.

Primary foods or positive foods

All vegetables and fruits of the concerned season (and not cold-storage ones) come under this category. These are called positive foods as these have a positive health value for the human being. These are also called primary foods because from the health point of view the intake of these foods assumes primary importance. Vegetables are subdivided into three sub-categories: (1) leafy vegetables, (2) non-leafy green vegetables, and (3) root vegetables; the non starchy ones like carrot, radish, beetroot being of a slightly superior order to the extent that these can be deemed to be equal to the non-leafy green vegetables from the viewpoint of nutrition. The starchy ones like potatoes, sweet potatoes, etc. are apparently vegetables in form but similar to cereals.

Such of the vegetables as could be taken raw or uncooked are best taken in that form. Take such vegetables, cut them or grate them along with the outer skin (which incidentally contain the maximum nutrients of the vegetable). Mix two, three or four of them in one plate but add no salt to them. Remember that the mineral salts, which are most needed by man for health, are in these vegetables and that these are the salts required by man. What is known as common salt available from the provision stores is not a plant product and is not really speaking needed by man from the viewpoint of nutrition. The moment some of the common salt is sprayed on the cut or grated vegetable, the latter will 'bleed' – their vital juices, will be drawn away. Nutritionally such salted vegetables are very, very inferior.

As many of the vegetables in the modern days happen to be grown on soil with chemical manures which literally rob the soil and upset the soil health happen to have lost their natural taste. They also happen to have lost much of the the normal nutrients that ought to be in these vegetables. To offset this serious deficiency I would suggest addition of grated coconut to the raw salad. Grated raw coconut incidentally contains practically all the vitamins and mineral salts. This is very tasty and addition of this will enrich the raw salad. Where available, fresh coriander leaves and tomato can be added to the raw vegetable.

The salad prepared thus should be consumed immediately after it is got ready. The roughage in this raw salad, especially the roughage from the grated coconut, would ensure easy and smooth passage of food from one end of the digestive canal to the other. And this roughage would enable man to maintain his bowel health in near ideal condition so that he can be free from constipation.

Let a good portion of your food be of this category, chew it thoroughly to ensure ideal digestion, be a vegetablarian, that is, one whose daily intake of food contains as much as 70 or 80 per cent of vegetables (raw and cooked combined). Mere vegetarianism is not enough; hence be a vegetablarian.

Where the vegetables cannot be taken raw, there can be no great harm in cooking them. Let them not be fried. Let them be steamed in a cooker, preferably a stainless steel cooker. Here again, first wash the whole vegetables, then cut them or grate them with their skin and put them in the cooker without adding any salt, condiments or spices at this stage. Let the vegetables (two or more can be cooked at the same time mixed together) be cooked in the cooker and as soon as the cooking is over, bring the cooker down. Open the lid a few minutes later and add to such cooked vegetables fresh coriander leaves, cut tomatoes and raw grated coconut. Add a little salt just to the extent needed and some condiments and spices, preferably of the less irritant type to the extent needed.

No frying is needed here; no need to add any pulses to the cooked vegetable as grated coconut contains the requisite proteins of the complete variety. No *ghee* either need be added at the end as grated coconut is there. Such conservatively cooked vegetable should be consumed as quickly as possible after cooking.

The moment the cooking process is over, the cooked stuff starts undergoing nutritional changes. When a cooked vegetable is taken one, two or three hours after cooking, much of the nutrients in it would have been lost. Hence taking cooked food immediately after cooking, as early as possible, is recommended.

Vegetable juices as food supplements will be of great value, especially to persons suffering from chronic and destructive diseases. Though the first one which I am going to mention is not actually vegetable juice, this is actually the best among the lot and hence requires mentioning at the top. This is the tender coconut water, which reaches the consumer straight from the producer, that is, the coconut tree in the same form, untampered in any way. Where available, the tender coconut water can be taken once early in the morning and the other in the late afternoon.

Any raw vegetable of the season from which juices cannot be extracted easily can be used as such, especially the leafy vegetables. Do not add any salt or any other seasoning.

The raw vegetable juices are to be sipped slowly and not gulped down the throat. No salt or sugar is to be added to them. These vegetable juices contain very many essential nutrients and being in the liquid form are easily assimilated in the human body. Notable among these are the raw juices of ash-gourd, the plantain pith, curry leaves (known in Hindi as *kari patta*), and the 'dhurva' grass.

Quite some people have to live at places where no fresh green vegetable is available for months on end. The leafy vegetables of the season available locally may be had in fairly good quantity (8 to 10 kilos)–two or three leafy vegetables can be mixed together–and these should be dried in shade so that the greenness of the leaves (known as chlorophyll) may not be lost. Within two or three day's time the leafy vegetables get dried. Get them together, powder them, bottle them and use when required. Such herbal powder can be of a great help. We can take a small quantity of it, mix it in water and drink; or alternatively we can add this herbal powder to the wheat flour *atta* and make *chapati*, which would be nutritionally better than the ordinary one.

Ideally speaking, fruits ought to be better than vegetables from the viewpoint of nutrition. But the methods adopted in modern days by fruit growers and fruit-sellers make the fruits more or less valueless. Most fruits are ripened overnight through chemicals, just within a few hours. It is a fact fairly well known that many of the chemicals are carcinogens, that is, capable of producing cancer. Again many of the fruits are produced far, far away. They are packed in wooden crates. Insecticides and pesticides are sprayed over them and when they reach the market located far away from the producing centre for being sold locally, their health value is 'more on the negative side'. For those who live in big cities and towns, including the adjoining villages, this sorry state of affairs is there to face. Hence here is a caution for the health-seekers. Use only seasonal fruits and not cold storage ones. From among the fruits available locally, there may be a few which are not ripened overnight through chemicals and on which spraying of insecticides and pesticides may be the least or may not be there. As far as is known to the writer, such fruits are guava, pears, fruits of the melon variety, oranges or *mosambee*, pineapple. As per the season, take whatever is available to you.

If anyone happens to live completely in rural surroundings, the problem mentioned here may not arise and good fruits may be available to such persons.

Where needed, prepare the fruit juices personally at home and consume them quickly. But never go in for tinned or bottled juices as these generally contain synthetic colours, synthetic flavours and even synthetic glucose. These also contain preservatives.

Secondary or negative foods

These are called secondary foods as they are not as essential to man's health as primary foods are. These are grains, all cereals like rice, wheat, millets like maize, *bajra*, etc., pulses and grams, milk and milk products. Even milk is secondary to man, as it can only be primary for the young ones of the cow or the buffalo. These foods predominate either in starch and/or proteins and/or fat. These cannot be digested as easily as the primary foods and these contain, comparatively speaking, far less vitamins, minerals, enzymes, etc.

There is one great danger in regard to these foods. Practically none of them is available to the consumer in its natural form. Rice is polished, the bran of wheat is removed in milling, the outer covering of pulses and grams are removed and even milk is available to consumer hours after milking in a pasteurised form. In the form these foods are available to most men and women in the modern days, these foods are far from ideal.

Ideally speaking hand-pounded rice, hand-ground wheat flour, pulses with their outer coverings intact and fresh milk as given by the cow/buffalo (within two or three hours of milking) are the ideal ones. Even where such ideal foods are available, they are of the secondary variety. But where they are not available even in this form, their use can impair health. Hence all health-seekers are advised to slash down their intake of these secondary foods to the greatest extent possible. No harm will result to them if they take grated coconut along with raw and steamed vegetables every day. People who can financially afford, can take almond, cashew nut and such other natural nuts unsalted, unfried, but in a small quantity.

Here too, avoid the use of oil, *ghee,* etc. for frying in any form as fried foods are to be deemed equal to 'burnt currency notes'.

Let the preparation of *chapati*, rice, bread be in tune with the principles of natural hygiene and let these be consumed in as small a quantity as possible.

While vegetables and fruits in their natural form are highly alkaline in nature, secondary foods are only neutral foods. But when the latter are perverted, they turn predominantly acidic. Foods of the third variety, devitalised foods, are also predominantly acidic. Let this caution be borne in mind.

Denatured or devitalising foods

A brief mention of these has been made earlier in this chapter. To the extent the man has taken any of these, he would be taxing his vitality. But he will not be able to gain any nutrition out of it. The chemicals, preservatives, etc. in most of these products are likely to harm the health of man. As these are not at all needed, I am not dealing with them *in extenso* here.

Eat frugally and chew thoroughly

What is good for health-maintenance/ health-restoration should be clearly understood by every health-seeker. Eat frugally. Never fill up the stomach more than half its capacity. Sticking to this principle would ensure proper peristaltic activity and digestion by the stomach and hence of the small intestine too.

Avoid over-eating. Never take more than two meals a day. Chew every morsel of your food thoroughly to ensure good salivary digestion. If there is good salivary digestion, gastric digestion and intestinal digestion too would be good. Hence chew your food thoroughly, eat slowly.

On the one hand the food eaten by a person should be digested and assimilated by his organism, on the other, he has to ensure that enough biological rest is given to his digestive organs every day. To ensure this, the ideal thing is to take in only two meals a day — first somewhere about midday and the second fairly early at night before 8 or 8.30 p.m. As work and digestion go ill together, the day-meal ought to be fairly light so that the outward work to be done by the individual, mental or physical, does not disturb the digestive process. The day's work should be completed by 6 or 7 p.m. and the person should go home relaxed with the satisfaction that he had done full justice in his business/office. Based on the noble dictum 'work while you work, play while you play', the person should slip into his domestic kingdom, forgetting his official worries totally. Thus relaxed, he is expected to take his night meal moderately with plenty of raw and steamed vegetables; take a little stroll after the meal and go to bed thereafter.

Let it be remembered that no living being other than the human would work on a loaded stomach. Let not man violate this sacred rule.

As a rule man does not require any food early in the morning. But to pander to human weakness one could take in some fruit juice or a little vegetable juice or some tender coconut water in the morning. Nothing more is advisable (patients suffering from chronic and destructive diseases should scrupulously observe the 'no-breakfast plan' to obtain the maximum results from the other Nature cure applications that they may be adopting during the rest of the day).

When and when not to eat

To get the maximum results from the food eaten:

- Eat only when hungry.
- Eat after ensuring that you are free from tension or any other type of emotional upset or conflict.
- Eat only when you are sure that you can comfortably take physical rest for at least an-hour-and-half after the meal.
- Keep the mind cheerful and happy when eating.
- Eat only when you are not having any painful symptom anywhere in the body. Hence eating is to be avoided in all acute diseases.

Let each health-seeker plan his daily diet hygienically, unmindful of the blaring propaganda over the mass media around that such and such food supplies energy to the human body. Let the simple truth expounded in the rare ideal 'eat to live, not live to eat' be thoughtfully borne in mind all the time. If only the calorie theory of food has any meaning in it, it should be capable of disproving all what is told in almost every scripture of the world that life power (what is known as *prana shakti* in Indian philosophy) is what is keeping all beings alive in this world.

Hence the minimum requirement of food be taken in its natural form as designed by Nature, bearing in mind the principle of 'vital economy'. Where this principle is given the go by, there can be no question of the person's ability to enjoy physical health and mental health.

Occasional fasting

As there are several disturbing features adversely affecting man's health from outside, even the one who is carefully following the principles of natural hygiene will have to resort to occasional fasting. Fasting hygienically is the only way to ensure maintenance of health all through life.

Those who, because of their unawareness of the principles of natural hygiene, are now suffering from chronic or destructive diseases, should utilise the mode of fasting suited to their physical condition and recoup their heath slowly, steadily and judiciously. While the rest of the world is asserting that the term 'food' is synonymous with the term 'nutrition', we in natural hygiene point out that nutrition is the capacity of the living body to extract nutrients from food and that in order to improve the organism's capacity to derive nutrition from food everyone should keep up the structural integrity of all his organs and functional efficiency of all systems in proper tone — especially the tone of the digestive organs in the body. And let it be fully realised that sensible fasting off and on is the one sure way to keep the digestive system in tone. Fasting improves the man's ability to digest better and assimilate nutrients properly.

Anyone wanting to keep his digestion in order and also anyone who wants to radically regain his digestive tone should avoid the two major dietetic errors commonly committed by many in modern society:

- wrong modes of eating,
- wrong choice of foods.

The daily diet plan prevalent almost everywhere takes notice of neither of these errors. Even the so-called books on nutrition do not pointedly draw attention to the need for reforming the diet, avoiding the twin errors referred to. No wonder indigestion (in all its manifestations) and constipation are more the rule than the exception in modern society. It is only natural hygiene that urges the modern man to consume food in a manner wherein the digestive organs would not be taxed to even a small extent.

Wrong modes of eating involve

- Eating without hunger.
- Eating hurriedly without chewing.
- Eating more than twice a day.
- Eating foods in wrong combinations.
- Eating when one is emotionally upset.
- Eating just before commencing one's daily work (physical/mental).
- Eating in between work.

Natural hygiene gives positive hints to health-seekers on every one of these points.

Wrong choice of foods

This again is a point rarely taken into consideration in modern days. Here are instances indicating the wrong choice:

- Consuming refined, processed, manufactured, tinned, bottled, packed foods — all of which could be designated as foodless foods as these lack the needed vital nutrients and contain synthetic vitamins, synthetic minerals, synthetic colours, synthetic flavour, preservatives, etc. in them.

- Taking in very little vegetables or fruits in one's daily diet and confining the so-called meal to cereals and pulses.
- Taking in of cooked foods long after their preparation.
- Resorting to fried foods on the assumption that these are tastier.
- Using condiments and salt.
- Consuming cold-storage vegetables and fruits.
- Consuming milk and milk products under the impression that one is supplying proteins, fats, etc. to the body in good quantity — and this too of the pasteurised variety.
- Consuming eggs and flesh foods under the impression that these will 'strengthen' the body.

The four factors

Here are four vital factors that every health-seeker has to bear in mind when feeding himself. The four factors are:

- Wholeness
- Sun value or freshness factor
- Alkalinity
- Frugality

Wholeness factor: The plant kingdom produces every food product in a particular manner. Wisdom lies in taking these foods as given by the plants as whole as practicable.

Vegetables and fruits lose their freshness when these come from the cold storage. Only seasonal vegetables and fruits are to be consumed. These too have to be eaten with their skins on (except when this is impracticable), for, most of the vital nutrients are on these skins and the layers just below the skins. Again the vegetables and fruits are to be consumed soon after they are cut, sliced or grated, to avoid loss of nutrients through oxidation. Salt should not be sprayed over the cut vegetable/fruit as some vital nutrients like vitamin C are lost this way. Frying vegetables results in loss of practically all the nutrients in them.

Fruits artificially ripened (in just a few hours) through chemicals are very harmful to health. Such fruits cannot be considered as 'whole' or fresh. As for cereals and pulses, the minimum cooking that is needed to make them edible could, of course, be permitted. But such cooked foods have to be consumed within an hour or so of cooking. As for milk, where it is available fresh (i.e. drawn from the udder from cows hygienically cared for) could form a part of man's natural food. And even this should not be taken in within an hour or so of taking one's night meal or just an hour or so earlier before taking the morning meal. Ideally speaking such milk is to be consumed alone as it is only when the stomach is empty that it can secrete the enzyme known as rennin, that is very much needed to digest the milk.

Curds prepared out of fresh raw milk may be consumed in moderation but not after they have become sour in taste. To add sugar to curd in order to sweeten it would disturb the digestion of other foods too in the stomach.

While fresh butter/clarified butter (*ghee*) may be used in a very small quantity in the meal, oil/*ghee* applied profusely on foods would hinder gastric digestion.

The sun value or the freshness factor: So long as the vegetable/fruit is on the plant, its vital contact with its nourisher, the sun, is there. From the moment it is plucked out of the plant, it starts losing its freshness. The longer the time lag the more is the loss of taste and nutrients from the vegetables/fruits.

Even cereals and pulses in their uncooked form can keep their freshness only for a limited period. Thereafter the pulses start giving undesirable taste/odour.

Let every natural food be taken as fresh as could be possible to ensure that the eater gets 'sun value' from them.

The alkalinity factor: Here is a list of foods indicating whether they are predominantly alkaline, predominantly acidic or neutral. Based on this list let foods be taken raw, or conservatively cooked as may be needed, bearing in mind all the points discussed earlier.

Predominantly alkaline foods (in descending order)

- Leafy vegetables (the thinner the leaf the more alkaline it is)
(best)
- Non-leafy green vegetables
- Carrot, radish, etc. — root vegetables containing less of starch
- Potatoes, sweet potatoes, etc. — root vegetables containing more of starch comparatively
- Bran of hand-grounded wheat flour   (better)

Neutral foods (in descending order)

- Fresh hand-ground wheat flour with bran   (better)
- Fresh hand-pounded rice
- Fresh flattened rice
- Whole pulses (with husk)
- Dry fruits
- Fresh milk of healthy animals and the curd made therefrom
- Pure honey in very small quantity   (good)

Predominantly acidic foods (in ascending order)

- Fresh jaggery from palm   (good)
- Fresh jaggery from cane

- Wheat flour without bran
- Fresh, pure oil and clarified butter (*ghee*)
- Honey in more quantity
- Machine-pounded rice
- Stale curd and buttermilk
- De-husked pulses (washed)
- Pasteurised milk
- Eggs, flesh, fish, fowl, chicken
- White sugar
- Confectionery and sweets
- Cake, bakery products
- Hydrogenated oils   (bad)

The frugality factor: Not being misled by the conventional talks in the modern society let every health-seeker remember that the consumption of food has to be as frugal as may be needed. Let it be remembered that good digestion is possible when this factor is fully borne in mind while taking one's daily food. By sticking to this principle one will be practising the principle of 'vital economy' and the principle of 'non-violence' in his life enabling him to live long, to live healthy and to live purposefully.

Almost all books on modern nutrition contain balanced food charts directing man to consume, day after day, specified quantities of foods. The high calorie foods included in the charts/tables belong to the 'refined' quality. Again no thought is given to the individual limitation in the digestion of food or with various gradations in health level. As a natural hygienist, I would dismiss what all is given in these charts as irrational.

What is needed for maintenance of health, for improving one's health level progressively as also for regaining one's health back to normalcy is not the daily supply of the so-called balanced food (which is unbalanced in every way), but a balanced supply of all the basic needs of living in tune with the principles of 'vital economy' and principle of 'non-violence'. It is only this that could ensure maintenance of a high level of health.

Let there be no diet faddism. Let the total approach be adopted by everyone all through his life for ensuring health and longevity.

Let man's daily activities be all hygienically planned and gone through. But let no one be food conscious all the twenty-four hours of the day. Every one of the man's activities in life — physical and mental — has its share either in improving his health or in reducing his health. In other words, every activity of man has its share to contribute in relation to the maintenance of his health, the improvement of his health, the recovery of his health. Hence, let the total approach be adopted by every sincere health-seeker, for only this total approach can deliver the goods.

Ensuring Sound Constitution for the Progeny

There are ever so many factors influencing the happiness of the family. While each one of the factors may have its own importance, one very vital factor, which makes or mars the happiness of the family is the health of the children.

If by any chance even one child in the family happens to be ill for most of the time, the concerned elders can never be happy, however much financial resources or other facilities the family may be having. Hence, let every married couple straight from the time of their marriage take proper care to ensure that the child/children to be born to them would be healthy all through life. How to ensure it? Is this entirely in the hands of the married couple concerned? Let us delve into this matter in some depth.

The constitution is the physical frame endowed on the infant at the time of its birth. If the constitution so endowed on the child is sound, there would be no problem whatever in the proper development of the child on to adolescence and adulthood. If, on the other hand, an infant is born with poor constitution, it will be very difficult to make up for the deficiency later. Hence, stress is being laid on the observance on the part of the married couple on proper steps even before conception takes place and of the continued care endowed on the development of the foetus within the mother's womb till delivery takes place.

It is the male that provides the seed, the sperm. The female provides only boarding facilities for the growing foetus. Unless and until the female's reproductive system is healthy with her uterus in proper tone, it may be difficult for her to provide the boarding facilities and where the weakness of the female is considerable, there could even be either an abortion or a miscarriage

If the sperms in the seminal discharge of the male are not very fertile, even if conception takes place, the infant to be born might have a poor constitution. The problem gets worsened if the concerned female provides a little unhygienic attention to the growing foetus inside during her pregnancy. The poor constitution resulting from the weak sperms of the male will be worsened by the improper prenatal care by the concerned female and later (after the child's birth) by inadequate breast feeding.

Both the male and the female have their respective responsibilities in ensuring that the infant to be born has a sound constitution.

If a married couple indulges in frequent sexual activity, both the male and the female will weaken their respective reproductive systems. In the case of the male, the sperm will become less and less fertile. In the case of female, the pelvic congestion would progressively worsen with disorders concerning her menstruation.

A married couple can be happy and contented when the individual health of the husband and wife is near ideal. The woman is to the man what the banks are to a river. The reverse is also equally true. Let each one lead a regulated life. The self-regulation exercised by the husband and the wife is for the purpose of ensuring healthy offsprings with sound constitution in them. Let the actual sexual indulgence be as limited as possible. Let the male remember that every seminal discharge weakens his very nerve structure and may even weaken the brain (central nervous system) considerably, if there is excessive sexual indulgence over a period of time. In the case of a female, every sexual act shocks her nervous system, weakens her nerves and glands, adding to her pelvic congestion and consequent misery.

Remembering all the above facts, let the couple adopt self-control to the greatest extent possible. If such self-control is adopted both by the male and female understanding its significance and importance, their own physical health and mental health would improve tremendously and as and when conception takes place, there could be a healthy offspring with a sound constitution.

Self-control is not difficult to adopt while it is admitted that sex is an instinct, both in the male and female. It is not as if sensible control over the sex instinct cannot be exercised by the male/female. Much depends upon the kind of training, the type of education and the cultural practices current in the society. These shape the attitude of the young adult, male and female.

The so-called family planning methods advocated in the modern days appear to convey an impression to the young married couple that they can indulge to the extent they want and yet avoid conception. The object of limiting the number of children in the family may be achieved by these methods. But the 'licence' that these methods are giving to these married couples makes them lose their health considerably with the result that as and when conception takes place in a particular woman, a weakling is born, suffering all through its life with various diseases.

Wisdom decrees that we should plan for the birth of healthy children in every family — having sturdy constitution, brilliant intellect. This laudable object can never be achieved if the couple adopts methods advocated in the present society and dangled before the eyes of each couple. Let the present generation be careful to see that it is not accused by the future ones that it had misled humanity.

Let stress be on citizen planning, not simply limiting the pace of population growth.

The vexed question

The common man might well raise the question: "Is it possible for everyone to observe *brahmacharya*? Is not the sex instinct in the human being a powerful one, which can break all restrictions sought to be placed on them?"

What is advocated is not total *brahmacharya* but a modified *brahmacharya* for the married people. It is admitted that in modern times so many outside influences are there which make the human being more and more sexy. Much of the literature that is doled in the news-stands has sex as their main topic. The types of advertisements that are being released through the mass media are also on similar lines. The foodstuffs on the shelves in the market are denatured, devitalised, de-mineralised, many of them having chemical preservatives in them. To add to all these negative factors is the idea presented to the modern man that disease is inevitable in him and that whenever he has any distressing symptoms, he must take to the 'recognised' modes of treatment.

The combined result of all this is that barring a few, everyone else is weak and miserable with a weak nervous system and weak glandular system. In fact it would be said that such persons are existing and not living.

The type of modified *brahmacharya* that is recommended by the writer is the only sane and safe method if we want to build up a healthy society for the future. Our ideal should be — let every future generation be better in every way than the previous one, let there be progressive improvement. There is no alternative to this sensible suggestion. Let us not work towards total degeneration. Mankind has already before it the dangerous complaint of AIDS.

Can there be anything worse than this? Let all of us ponder over the matter, take a U-turn and work for progressive prosperity.

Hygienic living, the sole saviour

Those that see sense in the approach recommended above should take to natural hygiene and build up their physical and mental health. Quite some people may consider the adoption of natural hygiene as difficult but let them remember that to achieve the object of a progressively healthier generation, there is no other alternative.

If every married couple takes to hygienic living, maintenance of the modified *brahmacharya* approach recommended above would not be difficult to adopt. Thus citizen planning will be easy to achieve and the modern family planning methods can disappear from the scene.

Pe-natal care

The care endowed by the woman on the growing foetus all through pregnancy is what matters the most. Pregnancy is not a diseased condition. It does not require any so-called treatment. Let the pregnant woman feed herself sensibly, avoiding all overeating and wrong eating. Let all manufactured foods, processed foods and the like be kept away from the menu. Let food be eaten moderately. Let the diet be predominantly vegetarian with a good portion of it taken as raw salad sensibly prepared.

Let proper prenatal exercises be performed by every concerned woman to ensure that her pelvic muscles develop the strength needed by her. Let the woman concerned pay enough attention to her mental health and let her keep herself as calm as practicable.

Postnatal care

And, when after delivery, the woman concerned is blessed with a healthy child, with a sound constitution, let her remember that the infant on her lap would need to be cared for with all possible attention to ensure that she has enough breast milk (of good quality) for her infant. Let her stick to the vegetarian diet advocated earlier. The baby has to be kept on breastmilk alone (without anything from outside) for twelve months or at least for eight months. After eighth months, breast-feeding can be reduced to three per day and the child can be given some light fruit juice of seasonal fruits or tender coconut water. Water can be given at least once. After fifteen months the breast-feeding can be reduced to two and on other two occasions some soft fruits mashed properly could be given to the baby daily. And from 18th or 20th month, the mother's feeding can be reduced to one per day and the growing child can be given some thick vegetable soup, unsalted but with coconut milk added to it. By the time the child has passed the age of two, adult foods can be started in moderation and should be sensibly prepared.

During this postnatal stage the concerned woman should do the postnatal exercises to see that her reproductive system gets back into its proper shape.

A weak constitution cannot be toned up to any great extent through any known methods. Let the principles of hygienic living be adopted as they are the only reliable guide to ensure that the constitution is not weakened in any manner.

An infant born with a sound constitution can be weakened if the principles of hygienic living are violated. It would be difficult to rebuild the constitution back to its original stage. Hence, the only key to health is that hygienic living be adopted all the time.

A sound constitution is a basic need of living and let this not be denied to any child that is to be born.

Total Approach

Everyone in the world wants to enjoy ideal health but the fact remains that health appears to 'elude' most people. Why?

In the days of yore the man had no problems whatever. He took everything in the most natural form and his instincts guided him to eat only when he was hungry, to rest when he was tired, to keep away from strain and stress (which used to be rarely there) and to lead his life in an atmosphere where there were no man-made complications and problems. The situation today happens to be unfortunately at the other extreme. Man's natural instincts appear to have been by and large perverted. Air is polluted and water too. Tension which is a by-product of man's eagerness to take to high pressure living in tune with the urge of modern civilsation, the almost total absence of the need on man's part to have any worthwhile physical activity — these are only some, not all of puzzles and riddles created by man around him in the modern world. No wonder that diseases are rampant almost everywhere.

Here too, instead of tackling the real cause of disease, man goes on indulging in symptomatic treatment and 'corrective' surgery. Such is the dismal picture of man's health in modern days.

Quite a few persons here and there, who were earlier in the modern physician's regular nets, escape from it and take to natural hygiene for these see some ray of hope in this new approach. And these derive quite some benefits through the adoption of the new approach. But here too the snag is still there in very many cases. And, hence even those that adopt natural hygiene do not 'fully' benefit. Where lies this snag?

For centuries mankind had got addicted to the idea that the medicine man (who had mastered the art) is very necessary for curing a patient. Most of the fish that escape the net happen to run after a 'medicine man' here too. These consider that natural hygiene is an alternative system of medicine on par with other systems of medication. In other words, they do not recognise the truth fully and get into the clutches of some that dole out remedies of some type or the other — may be drugless — before them.

So long as this snag is there, there may be some little 'benefit' but the goal is yet far, far away.

So long as man happens to be remedy-minded and so long as he equates the apparent effect of a remedy with a radical cure of the original disease there is no hope for mankind. The fact that many people are taking to natural hygiene in modern days and even deriving some benefit out of it does not gladden the mind of the writer for practically everyone of these happens to be remedy-minded.

Psychologically speaking, the one who seeks remedies for his problems is an escapist inasmuch as he is unwilling to face his problem, to study his problem in depth and find the solution there-of by himself. And, a person who is possessed by this 'demon' of escapism does never, never recognise the truth and without recognising the truth no problem whatever can be solved.

Not an alternative system of medicine but...

Vested interests may crop up in every field. This was how the original *Ayurveda* which was in its pristine purity in ancient days in this country lost its lustre and has now become a glass piece (apparently shining).

Back in those earliest days when the population in the world used to be very, very sparse, man was living in isolated hamlets, huts and houses. Each one had to look after the satisfaction of all his needs, as there was no organised profession in the then society. And in the circumstances each one was caring for his own health. The science of *Ayurveda* in its pristine purity was there. Every one knew the basic concepts thereof and each one was his own doctor. The health problems were practically few.

What was the original *Ayurveda* that existed in those days? We may get an idea of it from the most ancient work *Ayurveda Sutram* (in Sanskrit). This rare work has been published by the University of Mysore and even now those having knowledge of Sanskrit might peruse the work. What has been told here is nothing other than natural hygiene, as we understand it today. How had perversion set in here? As, in course of time, the population began to grow and as man began to settle in small towns and villages, the need for creating some sort of occupational classification in society was felt. Various occupations, viz. of masons, carpenters, potters, teachers, etc. became established in society. The persons in each of these professions were serving the other people in exchange for the supply of their basic needs of living like foodgrains, clothes, etc. from others. This was a social development of the right type.

But a few people in society came up and said: "We shall be your doctors caring for your health and every one of you need not take the trouble of understanding *Ayurveda*." Society got divided into two groups: the medicine men and the others. In the initial stages no one was falling ill and hence the medicine men had no work whatever to do. Hence these began to make the science as complicated as possible and created an impression that everyone could not learn it. As time rolled by, more and more illnesses set in the society and *Ayurveda*, as is being practised today, is what has come out of this untoward development in society which started centuries ago.

Though lip service is being paid even these days to the words 'hygiene' and 'health', mankind as a whole seems to be in the dark and even those that have a knowledge of the science of Nature cure happen to present it as an alternative system of medicine in a little complicated manner for many of these happen to be professionals in their line — prototypes of those earliest *Ayurvedic* doctors who did not want all the people to be healthy but wanted patients to serve their (doctors') own ends.

What is popularly known as Nature cure is nothing other than what Acharya Lakshmana Sarma termed as 'life natural', the adoption of that mode of life as designed by Mother Nature. Some followers in the West term this as natural hygiene or the science of health based on Nature's laws of health which are eternal, inviolable and immutable. They could have called it simply 'hygiene' but to distinguish it from the spurious hygiene prevalent today using poisons and medicaments, the Westerners term it as natural hygiene.

Well man, your health totally depends upon your having a clean bloodstream, proper blood circulation with structural integrity of every organ within in its ideal or near ideal state and proper functional efficiency of every system (like the respiratory system, the digestive system, etc.) in good condition. Man, why not remind yourself of the truth that the conditions obtaining inside your body are entirely your own creation depending upon your habits of living? No one can make you ill if you are determined to be well and no one can give you health from outside if you are living wrongly. Why not remind yourself of these basic truths?

The above basic requirement of health can be had only if your body and mind are cared for as Nature intends you to care for them, for after all, the human body is designed by Nature and

Nature has complete suzerainty over all the functions and activities inside the organism. In other words, no mechanical manipulation from outside, no mechanical contrivances, etc. can help to 'normalise' the condition within.

Why not recognise this truth? Natural hygiene is a codification of the concerned natural laws of health. This is not an alternative system of medicine but a way of life to be followed by every sane and sensible person in the world.

Look, there is no alternative to natural hygiene. Do not consider this as an alternative system of medicine on par with the prevalent systems of medication to be resorted to when one is ill and to be given up when one is apparently well. In your own interest please take to natural hygiene as fish takes to water, understand the implications of natural hygiene to the fullest extent, adopt them in your daily life unmindful of the opinions of the people around. But for heaven's sake please adopt the total approach and not a fragmentary one.

Life power and vitality

The reputed saint who lived with us till very recently, Sri Aurbindo Ghose once said: "Living is experiencing the fullness of our being; all else is existence."

How many of us are experiencing this blissful state? Are not most in the modern world only existing? What can we do to have this experience during the lifetime of ours? The science of natural hygiene can practically help us for achieving the purpose in view. This science tells us in no uncertain terms that life power or *prana shakti* functioning in each living organism is a gift of Mother Nature to every one of us. This power cannot be had from anywhere else in the world and it is the most valuable possession of every living being as life depends upon it.

It is there in everyone of us, unknown to us, deep inside the living being somewhere hidden to us — as vital reserve. A very small part of it is given to us every morning for carrying on that day's activities in the world. And this is vitality or *jeevan shakti*. The science of natural hygiene firmly asserts that economising the expenditure of vitality is the only means for maintaining health and for regaining health. In fact our contention is that all medicaments (prescribed through various systems of medication ostensibly to cure patients) rob patients of their vitality and hence are totally unscientific.

If many modern men happen to suffer from chronic and destructive diseases it is because their lifestyles are such as leading to wastage of vitality in their day-to-day lives. Return to normalcy in such cases would be possible only when the wasteful practices stop, giving place to near-ideal living. This is the reason why we insist on the practice of 'vital economy' in daily life. This is why we appeal to patients to take to non-violent applications, as every violent application will lead to further enervation.

Thus the central core is 'vital economy'. In practicing this 'vital economy' in daily life we have to ensure the supply of the basic needs of living to the person in proper proportion.

The basic needs of living are:

(1) *Physical*: constitution, activity (function, exercise, work), structural integrity of organs, functional efficiency of the different systems, cool air, water, food, sunshine, sleep (relaxation, repose, rest), posture, cleanliness.

(2) *Mental*: integrity at mental level (clarity, character, positive attitude), activity (work), faith (in the fundamental goodness of Nature), proper attitude towards one's daily work, observance of orderliness and systematic discharge of work, happiness, etc.

A balanced supply of the basic needs of living is what is required to ensure normalcy of activity in the organism — this is what the word 'health' implies. Where due to imperfect understanding a person lays stress upon just two or three factors (e.g. proper food, the morning walk, exercise) and where consequently many other essential factors are not taken care of to the degree required, maintenance of/improvement in the health level cannot be had. And where some of the basic needs are not supplied to the extent required, even the observance of 'vital economy' would not be practicable. Hence, we insist on sufficient care being exercised by an individual to ensure that all basic needs of living are supplied in a balanced manner.

In modern days 'experts' in particular fields of knowledge tend to overemphasise misleading the health-seeker that their standpoint alone is very important if one wants to be healthy. For instance, an 'expert' on *yogasana* and *pranayama* says that regular performance of certain *yogasana* and *pranayama* are the only sine qua non of healthy life. Another expert stresses upon 'meditation'. A third says that food is all-important. The fourth one insists on just one point like chewing of food.

While what each one of the above is saying is correct, so far as it goes, the human tendency to neglect the other essential points would complicate matters and lead to ill-health in due course of time.

Let no one belong to the category of the six blind men (referred to in the story, *Six Blind Men and the Elephant*) each of whom insists that he alone is correct and the others are wrong, while the real fact is that no one had seen the whole elephant. Hence, my plea is that every health-seeker should adopt the total approach. Every health-seeker is expected to have an all-round approach on the subject of health maintenance/ health recovery. When such total approach is there in an individual, he would so order his daily life which will enable the establishment of orderliness within the organism.

Order and the Ordainer

Establishment of the order referred to above would set a person on progressive improvement in his health level and where such an order becomes an established practice in one's day-to-day life, the principle of 'vital economy' is observed to the nth degree. No organ could in those circumstances be subjected to any violence.

Everything in this world is going on in an orderly way. If man through his antics disturbs the balance in Nature, this order gets upset. The science of ecology recognises this fundamental truth and calls upon man not to indulge in his nefarious attempts to disturb this balance in Nature.

The disturbing features or disorders observed in the modern world are just man-made ones. Left to Nature, the order is maintained all through in all aspects.

With such order serving as the basis of the world's existence everywhere, the wise ones point out that the Ordainer is behind the whole order.

As the subject under discussion is man's health, the order that ought to be there inside the functioning of the different organs/ systems, the somatic awareness that ought to be there in every living cell of the human body, the symbiotic relationship that ought to be there among the different systems in the body, is all under the full control of life power, *prana shakti*, which is the Ordainer within.

The rather unfortunate fact that is present the world over of man's suffering from chronic and destructive diseases is primarily due to the meaningless waste of life power within in various ways, many of which are foisted on immature minds through what goes by the name of modern civilisation. Logic tells us that proper care exercised by man in redesigning his pattern of life would re-establish the order within and make him healthy.

Let the discerning individuals who can clearly differentiate between the chaff and the grain spurn away the chaff and by ensuring a balanced supply of the basic needs of living, put themselves on the path of health, progressively improving their health level as days go by. Let the subject of natural hygiene be studied in depth. Let the basic truth of this science be ever borne in mind and let life in this world be lived purposefully.

The holistic approach

As lack of any positive result through the different systems of medication is being experienced by more and more patients in the modern world, they switch over to Nature cure in the hope that the diseases could be cured thus.

As these persons take to Nature cure only as an alternative system of medicine, there are a number of healers ready to oblige them. Though the system is getting more and more popular, its real significance and objective are forgotten both by the practitioner and the patient. The practitioners are anxious to produce 'immediate results' and with this sole objective so many procedures are being adopted. Maybe that in these procedures no chemicals or poisons as such are being employed. On this ground the practitioners insist that every one of these new procedures should also form part of Nature cure approach to give the system a holistic colour.

The so-called holistic procedures recently introduced by many practitioners into the system of Nature cure and against which I raise my voice of protest are:

- Acupuncture
- Accupressure
- Electrotherapy
- Magnetotherapy

- Reflexotherapy   • Chromotherapy

The so-called *yogic kriyas* like the *kunjal, neti* (*jal, sutra, ghrit* included), *vasti kriya* and the *hathayogic* procedures, *pranayama* like *bhastrika, kapalbhati*, etc. far beyond the capacity of the modern man, especially by those suffering from chronic disease.

With nearly sixty years of experience in natural hygiene, I make bold to say that every one of the above procedures violate the law of cause and effect, the principle of 'vital economy' and the principle of 'non-violence', all of which have a great bearing on regaining health, retaining health and improving it progressively. Apart from the applications (therapies) listed above, many persons advocate the use of established sciences like palmistry, astrology, astronomy, etc. If we look into the original works (forming a part of our Vedic culture), I have all admiration for the saints and sages who had done intense internal research and presented them to humanity.

I should not, in the circumstances, object to the use of these. But one or two stray points taken out of these sciences by the opportunists (lacking a dedicated knowledge of the subject) are applied these days on patients for giving them immediate symptomatic relief. The patients take these procedures as remedies wherein the reverence to the original sciences is totally lost sight of. Any procedure adopted just as a remedy 'dealing with the present problem/issue' can never be holistic.

The term holistic is being used by all and sundry, practitioners and patients alike. While every one seems to be satisfied with this or that holistic procedure, no one seems to worry about the following major issues involved in 'polluting' the science of Nature cure:

- Do not let perversions thus introduced into the system of Nature cure go against the fundamental philosophy of this science?

- Do not let these procedures do violence on one or the other organ in the human body and as such are these not as bad as, if not worse than, drugs/chemicals advocated by the different medications?

- Does not everyone of these procedures occasion wastage of the 'vital power' in the organism?

- Does not everyone of these procedures act as a remedy for giving immediate symptomatic relief and thus is not application of these procedures against the law of cause and effect, a fundamental natural law characteristic of the approach advocated by the science of Nature cure?

- As patients adopting one or the other of these procedures would only be remedy minded, would they at all care to reform their diet or to change their earlier habits of living the hygienic way?

- As no disease can be radically cured without removing the basic cause thereof, these so-called holistic methods by occasioning immediate symptomatic relief to the patient make the patients forget their real duty to radically change their habits of living the hygienic way.

- Would not the application of these holistic procedures result in the loss of structural integrity of one or the other vital organ inside?

- Would not the application of these holistic procedures impair the functional efficiency of the different systems in the human organism?

To the practitioners and the patients alike I would pose a question before them: "In case your resorting to one or the other so-called holistic procedures is going to thwart the development of

Nature cure as a science, would you like to be party to this unprincipled and illogical development?"

Dear patients, you can have even immediate symptomatic relief without any of these holistic procedures and you will stand to fully benefit by adopting applications of basic Nature cure (which is but a synonym for natural hygiene).

Anyone wanting to benefit fully by following basic Nature cure should avoid mistaking the different applications in Nature cure as the only factors which could help in recovering from disease. Here is a fervent appeal by an ardent disciple of Acharya Lakshmana Sarma, who was compassion-incarnate, to adopt the total approach for achieving the noble objective before everyone of us. Better keep away from the fragmentary approach and take to total approach.